Well-being for Thoracic Surgeons

Editor

CHERIE P. ERKMEN

THORACIC SURGERY CLINICS

www.thoracic.theclinics.com

Consulting Editor
VIRGINIA R. LITLE

August 2024 • Volume 34 • Number 3

ELSEVIER

1600 John F. Kennedy Boulevard • Suite 1800 • Philadelphia, Pennsylvania, 19103-2899

http://www.thoracic.theclinics.com

THORACIC SURGERY CLINICS Volume 34, Number 3
August 2024 ISSN 1547-4127, ISBN-13: 978-0-443-24688-3

Editor: John Vassallo (j.vassallo@elsevier.com)
Developmental Editor: Anita Chamoli

Thoracic Surgery Clinics (ISSN 1547-4127) is published quarterly by Elsevier Inc., 360 Park Avenue South, New York, NY 10010-1710. Months of publication are February, May, August, and November. Business and editorial offices: 1600 John F. Kennedy Boulevard, Suite 1800, Philadelphia, PA 19103-2899. Periodicals postage paid at New York, NY, and additional mailing offices. Subscription prices are $434.00 per year (US individuals), $100.00 per year (US students), $487.00 per year (Canadian individuals), $100.00 per year (Canadian students), $225.00 per year (international students), $524.00 per year (international individuals). For institutional access pricing please contact Customer Service via the contact information below Foreign air speed delivery is included in all Clinics' subscription prices. All prices are subject to change without notice. **POSTMASTER:** Send address changes to Thoracic Surgery Clinics, Elsevier Health Sciences Division, Subscription Customer Service, 3251 Riverport Lane, Maryland Heights, MO 63043. **Customer Service (orders, claims, online, change of address): Telephone: 1-800-654-2452 (U.S. and Canada); 314-447-8871 (outside U.S. and Canada). Fax: 314-447-8029. E-mail: journalscustomerservice-u-sa@elsevier.com (for print support); journalsonlinesupport-usa@elsevier.com (for online support).**

Reprints. For copies of 100 or more, of articles in this publication, please contact Commercial Rights Department, Elsevier Inc., 360 Park Avenue South, New York, NY 10010-1710. Tel: 212-633-3874; Fax: 212-633-3820; E-mail: reprints@elsevier.com.

Thoracic Surgery Clinics is covered in *MEDLINE/PubMed (Index Medicus), EMBASE/Excerpta Medica, Science Citation Index Expanded (SciSearch®), Journal Citation Reports/Science Edition,* and *Current Contents®/Clinical Medicine.*

Contributors

CONSULTING EDITOR

VIRGINIA R. LITLE, MD
Chief of Thoracic Surgery, Steward Medical
Group Thoracic Surgery, Brighton,
Massachusetts, USA

EDITOR

CHERIE P. ERKMEN, MD
Professor, Center for Asian Health, Lewis Katz
School of Medicine at Temple University,
Professor of Thoracic Surgery, Founding
Program Director, Thoracic Surgery
Fellowship, Department of Thoracic Medicine
and Surgery, Temple University Hospital,
Philadelphia, Pennsylvania

AUTHORS

MARA B. ANTONOFF, MD
Associate Professor, Division of Surgery,
Department of Thoracic and Cardiovascular
Surgery, The University of Texas MD Anderson
Cancer Center, Houston, Texas

AZZAN N. ARIF, MD
Fellow, Division of Thoracic Surgery,
Department of Surgical Oncology, Fox Chase
Cancer Center, Temple University Health
Systems, Philadelphia, Pennsylvania

PARNIA BEHINAEIN, MS
Medical Student, School of Medicine, Wayne
State University, Detroit, Michigan

IAN C. BOSTOCK, MD, MS, FACS
Assistant Professor of Surgery, Department of
Cardiothoracic Surgery, Medical University of
South Carolina, Charleston, South Carolina

ROSS M. BREMNER, MD, PhD
Department Chair, Norton Thoracic Institute,
St. Joseph's Hospital and Medical Center,
School of Medicine, Creighton University,
Phoenix Health Sciences Campus, Phoenix,
Arizona

ANDREA J. CARPENTER, MD, PhD
Assistant Dean for Health Systems Science,
Professor, Department of Cardiothoracic
Surgery, Joe R. and Teresa Lozano
Long School of Medicine, San Antonio,
Texas

LOUIS F. CHAI, MD
Thoracic Surgery Fellow, Department of
Thoracic Medicine and Surgery, Temple
University Hospital, Philadelphia,
Pennsylvania

NICOLAS CONTRERAS, MD
Assistant Professor of Surgery, Cardiothoracic
Surgeon, Division of Cardiothoracic Surgery,
University of Utah, Huntsman Cancer Institute,
Salt Lake City, Utah

CHERIE P. ERKMEN, MD
Professor, Center for Asian Health, Lewis Katz
School of Medicine at Temple University,
Professor of Thoracic Surgery, Founding
Program Director, Thoracic Surgery
Fellowship, Department of Thoracic Medicine
and Surgery, Temple University Hospital,
Philadelphia, Pennsylvania

JAIRO ANDRES ESPINOSA, MD
Cardiothoracic Surgeon, Southern
California Heart Centers, San Gabriel,
California

RACHAEL ESSIG, MD
Resident Physician, Department of Surgery, Georgetown University Hospital, Washington, DC

SHUBHAM GULATI, MS
Medical Student, Icahn School of Medicine at Mount Sinai, Mount Sinai Health System, New York, New York; Research Trainee, Division of Thoracic Surgery, Brigham and Women's Hospital, Harvard Medical School, Boston, Massachusetts

DAWN S. HUI, MD
Associate Professor, Department of Cardiothoracic Surgery, Joe R. and Teresa Lozano Long School of Medicine, San Antonio, Texas

HOLLIS HUTCHINGS, MD
General Surgery Resident, Henry Ford Health, Detroit, Michigan

CHI-FU JEFFREY YANG, MD
Associate Professor, Division of Thoracic Surgery, Department of Surgery, Massachusetts General Hospital, Boston, Massachusetts

KORIE CANDIS JONES-UNGERLEIDER, MD
Division of Cardiac Surgery, University of Michigan Medical Center, Ann Arbor, Michigan

MICHAEL MADDAUS, MD
Professor, Department of Surgery, University of Minnesota, Minneapolis, Minnesota

JESSICA MAGARINOS, MD
Resident Physician, Department of Surgery, Temple University, Philadelphia, Pennsylvania

M. BLAIR MARSHALL, MD
Director of Thoracic Oncology, Cardiothoracic Surgeon, Division of Thoracic Surgery, Sarasota Memorial Hospital, Sarasota, Florida

JOSEPH M. OBEID, MD
Cardiothoracic Surgery Fellow, Department of Cardiothoracic Surgery, Temple University Hospital, Philadelphia, Pennsylvania

IKENNA OKEREKE, MD
Vice Chairman, Professor, Department of Surgery, System Director, Thoracic Surgery, Michigan State University, Henry Ford Health System, Detroit, Michigan

ANNA OLDS, MD
Integrated Cardiothoracic Surgery Resident, Department of Surgery, University of Southern California, Los Angeles, California

AUNDREA OLIVER, MD
Associate Professor, Department of Cardiovascular Sciences, East Carolina Heart Institute, Eastern Carolina University, Greenville, North Carolina

SARA PEREIRA, MD
Professor, Division of Cardiothoracic Surgery, Department of Surgery, University of Utah, Salt Lake City, Utah

ALEXANDRA L. POTTER, BS
Research Assistant, Department of Surgery, Massachusetts General Hospital, Boston, Massachusetts

JOHN K. SADEGHI, MD
Cardiothoracic Surgery Fellow, Department of Cardiothoracic Surgery, Temple University Hospital, Philadelphia, Pennsylvania

MICHAEL P. SALNA, MD, MBA
Cardiothoracic Surgery Resident, Division of Cardiac, Thoracic, and Vascular Surgery, Department of Surgery, Columbia University Medical Center, New York, New York

BRYAN PAYNE STANIFER, MD, MPH
Assistant Professor, Division of Cardiac, Thoracic, and Vascular Surgery, Department of Surgery, Columbia University Medical Center, New York, New York

ANASTASIIA TOMPKINS, BS, BA
Research Associate, Center for Asian Health, Lewis Katz School of Medicine at Temple University, Philadelphia, Pennsylvania

GRAHAM DICKEY UNGERLEIDER, MD
Institute for Integrated Life Skills, LLC., Bermuda Run, North Carolina

JAMIE DICKEY UNGERLEIDER, MSW, PhD
Institute for Integrated Life Skills, LLC., Bermuda Run, North Carolina

ROSS M. UNGERLEIDER, MD, MBA
Co-Director, Institute for Integrated Life Skills, LLC., Bermuda Run, North Carolina

SHIVAEK VENKATESWARAN
Student, Research Assistant, Department of
Surgery, Massachusetts General Hospital,
Boston, Massachusetts

DUSTIN M. WALTERS, MD
Chief of Thoracic Surgery, Department of
Surgery, University of Connecticut,
Farmington, Connecticut

DANNY WANG, MD
Surgery Resident, Department of Surgery,
Massachusetts General Hospital, Boston,
Massachusetts

ANDREA S. WOLF, MD, MPH
Associate Professor, Department of Thoracic
Surgery, New York Mesothelioma Program,
The Icahn School of Medicine at Mount Sinai,
New York, New York

Contents

Cardiothoracic surgery, demanding in nature, often results in surgeons suffering from musculoskeletal injuries, causing chronic pain and leading to premature retirement. A significant majority report experiencing pain, exacerbated by minimally invasive techniques such as video-assisted thoracoscopic surgery. Despite this, many surgeons delay seeking medical assistance. To mitigate these risks, preventative strategies such as strength exercises, stretching during operations, and taking brief breaks are crucial. However, the surgical community faces a shortage of institutional support and comprehensive ergonomic education. Advancements in technology, including artificial intelligence and virtual reality, could offer future solutions.

Surgery of the chest is high stakes, and adverse events are common. Given the frequency and severity of such complications, cardiothoracic surgeons are at particularly high risk of becoming *second victims.* Even though our primary commitment as doctors is to take care of our patients, surgeons may fall into the emotional and intellectual trap of taking on the whole responsibility of a patient's poor outcome. This viewpoint may lead the physician to develop a heightened self-doubt, greater insecurity, and imposter syndrome, further affecting their ability to prevent complications and tackle difficult cases in the future.

Cardiothoracic surgeons work in high-intensity environments starting in surgical training and throughout their careers. They deal with critical patients. Their routine procedures are delicate, require extensive attention to detail, and can have detrimental effects on patients' lives. Cardiothoracic surgeons are required to perform at their best capacity incessantly. To do this, they must safeguard their mental and physical well-being. Preserving health through sleep, nutrition, exercise, and routine medical checkups ensures a cardiothoracic surgeon's well-being. Great personal effort and discipline is required to maintain health in a busy schedule. We offer our best recommendations from expert peers in the field.

of identifying themes within the workplace to strengthen camaraderie, minimize burnout, and enhance patient care. Key points highlighted include the vital role of teamwork and communication in providing safe and effective patient care. Various studies and initiatives underline the impact of improved teamwork and communication on reducing errors in health care settings.

THORACIC SURGERY CLINICS

Foreword
The Holistic Well of Being—
Let the Cup Runneth Over

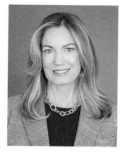

Virginia R. Litle, MD
Consulting Editor

Sometimes we need to put ourselves first to successfully apply what we signed up for: caring for others. We didn't choose this path because we are masochists. We chose it for the intellectual challenges and the passion for taking care of people. Just as we must be open to evolving technically, we must also be open to evolving personally. This issue of *Thoracic Surgery Clinics* entitled "Well-Being for Thoracic Surgeons" is guest edited by Dr Cherie P. Erkmen, who offers a detailed compendium of every personal facet of life we should stop and reexamine. How do we optimize our professional journey and not trip and fall over the frequent stress barriers innate to our practice? We build a "Resilience Bank Account" as summarized in Drs Dustin Walters' and Michael Maddaus' contribution "Strategies of Well-Being Training and Resilience," so we may be our best selves.

The postgraduate cardiothoracic training privileged us to practice one of the more complex areas of medicine. We improve societal health, but, ironically, we have fallen into unhealthy lifestyles and are at risk of cardiovascular disease, obesity, substance use disorders, and even suicidal ideation. The professional societies, including the Accreditation Council for Graduate Medical Education (ACGME), are taking baby steps to address these serious problems, and the history is summarized in the contribution by Dr Anna Olds and coauthors. When you think about it, the problem could be considered a public health crisis.

Our practices evolve technically, but they must also change in other spaces that have historically seemed soft to us—taking care of ourselves. Eat, sleep, and exercise are championed by Drs Andrea Wolf and Ross Bremner, who chair the American Association for Thoracic Surgery (AATS) Well-being Committee. Don't undervalue sleep. We need to change the culture. You're up all-night operating? Ask a colleague to help with clinical care the next day or talk with your patient and reschedule elective cases. This is not easy, but it will be when the culture changes. We also need to improve operating room ergonomics. Dr David Sugarbaker was ahead of his time when as the 2014 President of AATS, his invited guest speaker presented incorporation of exercise breaks in the operating room. In this *Thoracic Surgery Clinics* issue, Dr Jeff Chang and colleagues discuss safety and optimizing ergonomics. How many surgeons do you know—and maybe yourself—have had cervical disc decompression? You don't have to build up to the five-hour plank (and try to break a Guiness record), but strengthening your core, being physically cognizant, and taking breaks are better for you (and your patients).

This entire issue should be a bible for how to reassess our professional and personal culture. As summer with family and relaxation are upon us, this is the time to reflect and appreciate what we have. As pointed out in Walters' and Maddaus' article, humans have an inherent need for community connection and belonging to positively impact

Thorac Surg Clin 34 (2024) xi–xii
https://doi.org/10.1016/j.thorsurg.2024.05.007
1547-4127/24/© 2024 Published by Elsevier Inc.

our overall persona. The contribution by Dr Jamie Ungerleider and family details the science behind relationships and appropriately reminds us of the value of personal relationships to our well-being. In the AATS wellness survey, 44% of CT surgeons reported seldom or never having had adequate time with family. If you have your own family, spending time together is an integral component of positive mental health and holistic wellness. Compartmentalizing time to focus on family and not be distracted by patient issues is difficult but necessary. We are trained to put work first, as patients get sick 24/7 not on a 9 to 5, weekday schedule. We must recognize that our professional partners are capable of taking care of problems, and when we are off, the patients are not drifting aimlessly at sea. The culture of training and then practicing needs to evolve.

Thank you to our guest editor Dr Erkmen, and to all of the experts for their engaging submissions. Please read and *enjoy* this holistic issue of *Thoracic Surgery Clinics*.

Sincerely,

Virginia R. Litle, MD
St. Elizabeth's Medical Center
736 Cambridge Street
Cambridge, MA 02135, USA

E-mail address:
Vlitle@gmail.com

Twitter: @vlitlemd (V.R. Litle)

Preface

Shifting Paradigm from Achievement to Well-Being in Cardiothoracic Surgery

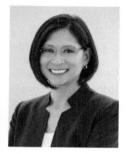

Cherie P. Erkmen, MD
Editor

Cardiothoracic surgeons are trained to manage disease processes of their patients. However, we do not receive training regarding management of our own well-being. In fact, surgeons have a long history of prioritizing service to others over personal well-being. William Stewart Halstead,[1] an icon of American surgery, developed our current principles of surgical training, anesthesia, and antiseptic technique. However, he and his career suffered from addiction to a precursor of cocaine and morphine. Cardiothoracic training, learned from icons and mentors of surgery, focuses on achievements and milestones, but not necessarily on well-being. Though difficult to define, well-being is the sum state derived from positive physical, mental, social, and environmental experiences.[2]

Well-being is a critical priority for cardiothoracic surgeons. Our profession faces challenges of increasing complexity of patient management paradigms, integration of rapidly expanding technology, and financial constraints. We have responsibilities to our patients, colleagues, trainees, family, and friends. Furthermore, a shortage of cardiothoracic surgeons will compel a 121% increased workload for each cardiothoracic surgeon by 2035.[3]

The only way to meet these challenges is to ensure peak performance and longevity of each cardiothoracic surgeon. We must eschew the oversimplified concept of achieving work-life balance, which suggests that prioritizing one causes sacrifice of the other. The shifting paradigm is to strive for well-being across all domains of one's life. Evidence-based principles for achieving well-being among cardiothoracic surgeons include striving toward a goal, work commensurate with goals, interconnectedness with others, social relatedness to work, a culture of safety and autonomy.[2] With this issue, we develop these principles with practical applications to a career in cardiothoracic surgery. Though each article is an independent review of an aspect of well-being, they are all interconnected (**Fig. 1**). Questions or curiosities raised by one article will likely be addressed by other articles. Our hope is that this work will provide a foundation for continued learning and practice of well-being. By strengthening our skills of well-being, we will improve our own performance, thus enhancing our success with family, colleagues, trainees, patients, and our communities.

I thank our contributing authors, who have circumscribed challenging concepts into practical and relevant applications of well-being. I am indebted to Dr Virginia Litle and John Vassallo for their support of this unique work. I thank the staff of Elsevier, especially Anita Chamoli, who has guided all our authors with skill and kindness. It

Thorac Surg Clin 34 (2024) xiii–xiv
https://doi.org/10.1016/j.thorsurg.2024.05.001
1547-4127/24/© 2024 Published by Elsevier Inc.

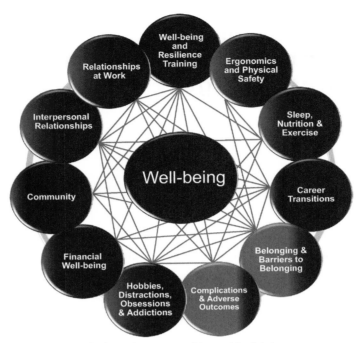

Fig. 1. Domains of well-being in cardiothoracic surgery addressed in this issue.

is my honor to have the opportunity to address this most critical topic of well-being.

Cherie P. Erkmen, MD
Department of Thoracic Medicine & Surgery
Temple University Hospital
Center for Asian Health
Lewis Katz School of Medicine at
Temple University
Thoracic Surgery
Temple University Health System
Suite 501 Parkinson Pavilion
3401 North Broad Street
Philadelphia, PA 19140, USA

E-mail address:
Cherie.P.Erkmen@tuhs.temple.edu

REFERENCES

1. Osborne MP. William Stewart Halsted: his life and contributions to surgery. Lancet Oncol 2007;8(3):256–65. https://doi.org/10.1016/S1470-2045(07)70076-1 PMID: 17329196.
2. Khalil S, Olds A, Chin K, Erkmen CP. Implementation of well-being for cardiothoracic surgeons. Thorac Surg Clin 2024;34(1):63–76. https://doi.org/10.1016/j.thorsurg.2023.08.006 Epub 2023 Oct 14. PMID: 37953054.
3. Moffatt-Bruce S, Crestanello J, Way DP, et al. Providing cardiothoracic services in 2035: signs of trouble ahead. J Thorac Cardiovasc Surg 2018; 155(2):824–9. https://doi.org/10.1016/j.jtcvs.2017.09.135 Epub 2017 Oct 31. PMID: 29221739.

Safety and Optimizing Ergonomics for Cardiothoracic Surgeons

Shivaek Venkateswaran[a], Danny Wang, MD[a], Alexandra L. Potter, BS[a], Chi-Fu Jeffrey Yang, MD[b],*

KEYWORDS

- Cardiothoracic surgery • Ergonomics • Work-related musculoskeletal disorder
- Minimally invasive surgery • Pain management

KEY POINTS

- Cardiothoracic surgeons face high rates of musculoskeletal injuries due to the demands of their surgical procedures.
- Many surgeons are hesitant to seek treatment for their musculoskeletal disorders, leading to aggravated conditions and affecting career longevity.
- Implementing preventative measures and mitigation strategies is crucial to minimize the risk of injuries in cardiothoracic surgery.

INTRODUCTION

Cardiothoracic surgery is a field known for requiring meticulous precision and immaculate technique that is equally physically demanding on its practitioners.[1] Cardiothoracic (CT) surgeons often spend long hours in the operating room (OR) in uncomfortable and unnatural positions resulting in physical wear and tear.[2,3] Over the lifetime of a surgeon's career, this can lead to permanent musculoskeletal injury, lifelong pain, and even early retirement, so much so that the prevalence of work-related musculoskeletal disorders among surgeons is often comparable to that of industrial workers.[4] Increasing awareness of ergonomics and preventative measures in the OR and workplace may prevent debilitating and career-ending injuries.[5]

Traditionally, surgical ergonomics in the OR has been overlooked and unsurprisingly a high prevalence of musculoskeletal pain and injury exists among surgeons. Studies suggest that roughly 66% to 94% of surgeons performing open surgeries and between 23% and 80% of robotic-assisted surgeries have experienced musculoskeletal pain at some point in their career[6] with one study finding 60% of surgeons reporting neck pain, 52% of surgeons reporting shoulder pain, and 49% of surgeons reporting back pain during a 12 month period.[7]

In a national survey of 600 CT surgeons, conducted by Mathey-Andrews and colleagues,[8] 64% of CT surgeons reported that they had experienced some type of musculoskeletal injury, which is consistent with previous studies; 35% of respondents indicated some degree of cervical spine injury which was the most commonly reported injury.[8] This was followed closely by lumbar spine injuries which affected 30% of respondents.[8] In multivariable adjusted analysis, cardiac surgeons were found to be more likely than thoracic surgeons to experience occupation-related musculoskeletal injuries.[8]

[a] Department of Surgery, Massachusetts General Hospital, 55 Fruit Street, Boston, MA 02114, USA; [b] Division of Thoracic Surgery, Department of Surgery, Massachusetts General Hospital, 55 Fruit Street, Boston, MA 02114, USA
* Corresponding author.
E-mail address: cjyang@mgh.harvard.edu

Thorac Surg Clin 34 (2024) 197–205
https://doi.org/10.1016/j.thorsurg.2024.04.007
1547-4127/24/© 2024 Elsevier Inc. All rights reserved.

The advent of minimally invasive surgery has also increased the physical demands of surgery. Video-assisted thoracoscopic surgery (VATS) and other minimally invasive approaches in general often require twisting and awkward maneuvers that generate undue stress on the surgeon's body.[9] A meta-analysis of surgical ergonomics published by Stucky and colleagues[10] found that surgeons who predominantly perform minimally invasive surgery were more likely to experience neck, arm/shoulder, hand, and leg pain as well as higher odds of fatigue and numbness than surgeons performing predominantly open surgery. These results are corroborated by other studies with another review finding that musculoskeletal disorder rates for conventional laparoscopists range from 73% to 100%.[6] Although the minimally invasive approach to surgery is associated with improved patient outcomes and recovery,[11,12] this approach has presented new physical challenges to the surgeon.

Surgeons often do not reach out for help for their musculoskeletal issues. In one study, only 29% of surgeons took some measures to seek medical attention for their musculoskeletal pain[10] with another study finding that the majority (65%) never seeks out any help or advice for their pain.[13] Among cardiothoracic surgeons, even fewer are willing to report their symptoms, with only 12% of cardiothoracic surgeons with musculoskeletal pain willing to report their symptoms to their institution.[8] The strenuous nature of cardiothoracic surgery and general unwillingness to seek treatment or help for musculoskeletal issues results in festering injuries and lifelong pain.[14]

The impact of musculoskeletal injuries on a surgeon's health and practice has far-reaching consequences on their wellness and career. One meta-analysis of 21 articles spanning 5828 surgeons found that 12% of surgeons experiencing a musculoskeletal injury required a leave of absence or an early retirement.[7] This trend is exacerbated in CT surgery, where a national survey reported that 30% of CT surgeons experiencing musculoskeletal injuries took time away from work.[8] Of these surgeons who reported having to take time away, 23% ended up retiring early and among CT surgeons who retired early in general, and 55% reported retiring over a decade earlier than expected due to their musculoskeletal injury.[8] However, only 35% believed that the CT surgery community was supportive of applying ergonomics techniques in the OR.[8] Many studies have found that surgeons feel unsupported by their institutions and these studies have reported that there is generally a lack of adequate resources and education on the topic of ergonomics and musculoskeletal injury in surgery departments and hospitals[9,15,16]; clearly, this is a systemic issue that spans beyond just the OR. Especially amidst a shortage of cardiothoracic surgeons,[17] there is a critical need to protect and maintain the health and careers of cardiothoracic surgeons.[18]

DISCUSSION
Preventative Measures

The demanding nature of cardiothoracic surgery necessitates a proactive approach to maintaining a surgeon's physical health and preventing musculoskeletal disorders. Strengthening exercises, intraoperative stretching, and microbreaks are beneficial strategies that promote physical resilience and reduce the risk of injury in the OR.

Strengthening Exercises

Cardiothoracic surgeons can benefit from a regular regimen of strength training tailored to the specific demands of surgical procedures. Focus should be on exercises that enhance core stability, upper body strength, and posture.[19] The implementation of a structured strength training program has shown promise in mitigating work-related musculoskeletal pain among surgeons.[5,20] Important exercises include deep cervical flexor training and standing scapular retraction[19] (**Fig. 1**).

These exercises can help to improve posture and reduce neck and upper back pain during tedious surgical procedures. To perform deep cervical flexor training, one should hold (or imagine holding if they are scrubbed) their closed fist between their chin and chest and flex their neck for 10 seconds.[19] During this, the engagement of the front neck muscles can be felt.[19] Repeating this 10 times throughout the day will result in increased strength.[19] To perform standing scapular retraction, one should pull their shoulder blades down and toward the spine, pulling their upper trapezius down away from the ceiling.[19] This position should be held for 5 to 10 seconds and repeat roughly 10 times daily for optimal results.[19,20] Additionally, core exercises such as planks and back extensions fortify the muscles used to maintain operative posture.[5,21] At the same time, targeted resistance training for the upper extremities can reduce the fatigue associated with prolonged surgical procedures and musculoskeletal pain.[5,21,22]

Intraoperative Stretching

Incorporating stretching into the surgical routine can also provide significant benefits.[19] Stretching exercises that target the neck, shoulders, and back, performed before and after operations, can improve circulation and alleviate tension that has

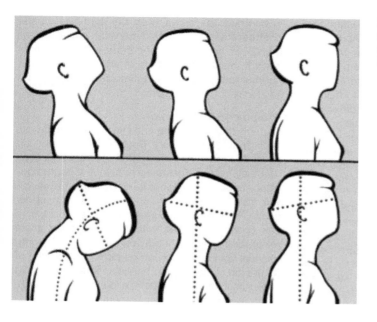

Fig. 1. Deep cervical flexor training diagram. (Lewit, K., Manipulative therapy: Musculoskeletal Medicine. 1st Edition, 2010, Churchill Livingstone.)

accumulated throughout an operation.[19] For example, cervical range of motion exercises can help reduce neck pain. In a national survey of 600 cardiothoracic surgeons, 45% of cardiac surgeons and 24% of thoracic surgeons experience cervical spine injuries.[8] Moving one's neck in each direction 10 times every 20 to 40 minutes or when experiencing stiffness in the neck can help reduce cervical pain.[19] Additionally, stretching the upper trapezius, levator scapulae, and pectoralis will improve upper neck and shoulder pain.[19] Dynamic stretches that simulate the body during surgery may acclimate the body to the demands of specific procedures, potentially reducing the incidence of overuse injuries.[19]

The American College of Surgeons' surgical ergonomics recommendations encompass a variety of dynamic exercises, including range of motion exercises for the neck (extension, flexion, and left/right rotation), cervical and shoulder stretches, and hand and elbow stretches.[19]

A randomized controlled clinical trial performed by Giagio and colleagues[23] investigated the impact that stretching can have on reducing work-related musculoskeletal disorders. Over a 6 month period, surgeons were randomized to a comprehensive "Preventative Program" ($n = 65$) or to no intervention ($n = 76$).[23] This preventative program placed an emphasis on instruction of ergonomics principles and prescribed a stretching regimen to surgeons under the supervision of a physical therapist.[23] Upon completion of the trial, surgeons in preventative program group saw significant improvement in their quality of life and

significant reduction of lower back pain after 3 and 6 months.[23] After 6 months, surgeons in the preventative program also saw a significant reduction in analgesic consumption indicating an overall reduction in pain after performing such exercises and stretches.[23]

Microbreaks

Microbreaks are brief pauses in the operative workflow that allow surgeons to reset their posture and perform light stretching techniques or relaxation techniques.[24] These short intervals, ranging from 30 seconds to a few minutes, can significantly reduce the static muscle load and mental fatigue associated with long operations.[24–26] One multi-institutional study instructed surgeons to take microbreaks every 20 to 40 minutes. This intervention resulted in improved pain reduction, physical performance, and mental focus. Afterward, 87% of surgeons in the study wanted to incorporate microbreaks into their OR routines.[26]

Mitigation Strategies

Mitigation strategies in the OR for cardiothoracic surgeons aim to optimize the environment, self, and equipment to reduce ergonomic strain and prevent musculoskeletal injuries.

Optimizing the Environment

Optimizing the environment is essential to ensure that surgeon health is preserved during the long hours spent in the OR. These principles are sparingly taught during training and are often neglected and not emphasized in practice.[27]

One example of such optimization is adjusting the operating table height. The table should be adjusted to maintain the surgeon's elbows at a 90° angle to prevent musculoskeletal strain during both open and minimally invasive procedures.[19] For open surgery, this is roughly elbow height, and for VATS, this is pubis height.[19] Another key environmental optimization is ensuring the appropriate monitor placement.[19] The monitor should be placed with the top of the screen at eye level and the center of the screen slightly below eye level, which helps maintain a neutral cervical position, which is vital to reducing neck strain.[19] These adjustments are supported by findings indicating that such environmental modifications can reduce the need for work leave and promote intraoperative adjustments that may prevent future complaints.[28,29] The use of anti-fatigue mats is recommended by many organizations such as the Occupational Safety and Health Administration (OSHA) and Canadian Centre for Occupational Health and Safety (CCOHS)[30,31] and supported by data.[32,33] However, some studies have questioned the effectiveness of anti-fatigue mats. For example, Voss and colleagues[3] evaluated the use of anti-fatigue mats for 175 oncological surgeons at MD Anderson and found that floor mat usage was associated with increased discomfort. Taking this into account, the usage of floor mats should be left up to the surgeon's discretion and comfort.[3]

Physical Optimization

Prolonged stance is an often overlooked contributor to musculoskeletal injuries. Simple maneuvers such as minimizing forward head posture can be of great benefit, as it is common in both open and minimally invasive cardiothoracic surgery. Although tilting the head forward an inch may not appear to make much difference, each inch of forward head posture can increase the effective weight of the head on the spine by an additional 10 pounds, underscoring the necessity to maintain a neutral neck position.[9] Forward head posture also leads to increased strain on the cervical and thoracic musculature, cervical disc problems (primarily C5–6, C6–7), tension headaches, increased neural tension of upper extremities, and loss of cervical and thoracic mobility.[34–37] Prolonged stance can exacerbate tension and can lead to chronic cervical pain, scapular pain, upper extremity paresthesia, and tension headaches.[38]

Fig. 2 shows 2 examples of surgeons, one with poor posture and one with optimal posture.

The first surgeon is hunched over the operating field, compromising his cervical and lumbar spine.

In contrast, the surgeon on the right has a safer posture and an improved cervical angle of less than 25°.[5] Additionally, she demonstrates a slight bend in her knees and equal weight distribution, another form of physical optimization that is beneficial in reducing leg pains.[5]

Equipment Optimization

Properly fitted equipment can vastly reduce the risk of musculoskeletal injury. Surgical equipment such as loupes must be fitted for the surgical field such that they allow surgeons to remain in a neutral position. Loupes that allow for angulation below 25° will also reduce strain on the neck and upper back.[39] Additionally, surgeons should be able to see under the lenses with the declination angle minimizing forward head posture and minimizing, cervical flexion, which can be common sources of neck pain.[5] If neck pain persists, surgeons should seek consultation to adjust the loupes' focal length.

For head-mounted equipment such as headlights, achieving an even weight distribution across the head is crucial. In procedures requiring fluoroscopy, two-piece lead vests are preferable to one-piece as they better distribute weight, reducing the risk of back strain.[40] Surgeons should also be prudent to remove these vests when they are not essential to the task at hand, preventing unnecessary physical burden.[41]

For VATS, instruments that allow for a neutral wrist grip, such as a pistol grip, should be selected.[42] Additionally, as noted in the "Optimizing the Environment" section, the VATS monitor should be placed on a boom that can be adjusted relative to the surgeon's height.[19]

Rehabilitation

If a cardiothoracic surgeon sustains an injury, effective rehabilitation strategies are pivotal to ensuring full recovery. The rehabilitation process for surgeons who have musculoskeletal disorders is multifaceted, emphasizing the importance of early intervention, comprehensive pain management, physical therapy, and psychological support.

The rehabilitation of surgeons who have musculoskeletal disorders hinges significantly on early intervention. In a randomized control trial conducted by Nordeman and colleagues,[43] it was confirmed that early access to physical therapy resulted in statistically greater improvement in pain than later access. With the data from this trial along with the conclusions of various other studies,[43–46] seeking interventions early can play a vital role in reducing pain and therefore prolonging a surgeon's career. Despite this, a national survey conducted by Mathey-Andrews and colleagues,[8] found that 97% of CT surgeons who

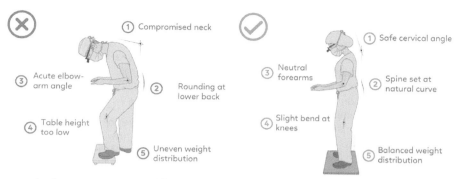

Fig. 2. Compromised surgeon posture with at-risk cervical and lumbar spine versus optimal surgeon posture. (*From*: Dairywala MI, Gupta S, Salna M, Nguyen TC. Surgeon Strength: Ergonomics and Strength Training in Cardiothoracic Surgery. Semin Thorac Cardiovasc Surg. Winter 2022;34(4):1220 to 1229. https://doi.org/10.1053/j.semtcvs.2021.09.015).

experienced work-related musculoskeletal injuries did not seek out an intervention for their injuries. These data also underscore the importance of early physical therapy as an effective and necessary treatment for CT surgeons after experiencing a work-related musculoskeletal disorder.

The national survey conducted by Mathey-Andrews and colleagues[8] concluded that the most common treatment among both cardiac and thoracic surgeons for musculoskeletal pain was non-narcotic analgesia. Unfortunately, approximately 13% of cardiac and 12% of thoracic surgeons have used narcotics to treat musculoskeletal pain in the past.[8] It is important to manage pain with multimodal analgesia and multidisciplinary approaches, including both pharmacologic and nonpharmacological therapies, to enhance recovery and improve quality of life.[47]

Supporting Surgeon's Mental Health

The psychological impact of musculoskeletal injuries caused by poor ergonomics is often overlooked and requires a multifaceted approach to rehabilitation. In a systematic review that looked at musculoskeletal sports injuries, Gennarelli and colleagues[48] found that psychosocial interventions, such as relaxation techniques, guided imagery, positive self-talk, and goal setting, significantly enhance recovery and pain management, which is particularly relevant for surgeons contending with the physical strains of their practice. Although this study is targeted toward athletes, the lessons learned from this study can be applied to cardiothoracic surgeons.[5,49] Furthermore, evidence shows that early psychosocial support can markedly improve quality of life and reduce psychiatric symptoms.[50] Importantly, the psychological impact of such injuries, often manifesting as depression, anxiety, and post-traumatic stress disorder (PTSD) symptoms, must be addressed promptly.[50]

Educational and Institutional Efforts

There is a striking gap in the provision of comprehensive surgical ergonomics education, which is essential for preventing work-related musculoskeletal disorders among surgeons. By exploring the current landscape of ergonomics education in the field of surgery, the challenges in implementing effective training programs, and the role of institutional support in ergonomic education, we can foster safer and more sustainable surgical practice.

The Necessity of Ergonomics Education

Despite such a high prevalence of work-related musculoskeletal disorders in surgery subspecialties across the board, there is an absence of dedicated surgical ergonomics education, with one survey by Epstein and colleagues[27] estimating that only 25.4% of surgeons have received surgical ergonomics education training and with only 1.5% of this group receiving education in a consistent fashion. The lack of ergonomics education goes beyond attending surgeons though, with a survey of all allopathic medical schools finding that 98% reported their students receiving less than three hours of ergonomics education.[51] Access to ergonomics education in residency programs is also minimal.[51] A study by Sergesketter and colleagues[52] found that roughly 75.3% of surveyed medical students reported musculoskeletal pain. These data suggest that there is an overarching problem of inadequate ergonomic training at multiple stages of medical and surgical education, which could even negatively impact on medical students' interest in surgical subspecialities which is especially concerning amidst a shortage of cardiothoracic surgeons.[17,18]

Current Educational Resources

Currently, one major resource for ergonomics education for surgeons is the American College of

Surgeons (ACS) Surgical Ergonomics Recommendations. Developed by the ACS Division of Education and its Surgical Ergonomics Committee, these recommendations are a comprehensive guide for surgeons. They are readily available for download and provide detailed advice on ergonomic practices in surgery.[19] ACS Division of Education and its Surgical Ergonomics Committee also host hands-on clinics for practicing surgeons and surgical trainees.[19] These clinics, such as the one held during the Annual Clinical Congress, provide practical training in surgical ergonomics.[19] The Society of Thoracic Surgeons also has implemented sessions on ergonomics during its annual meetings. Although these resources exist, institutions should also create their own resources tailored to the equipment and facilities in the hospital. Despite existing resources, the national survey conducted by Mathey-Andrews and colleagues[8] concluded that roughly 65% of cardiothoracic surgeons did not feel that the overall CT surgery community supported implementing ergonomic techniques, indicating that more needs to be done to promote education on surgical ergonomics.

Institutional Responsibility and Support

The alarming prevalence of occupational musculoskeletal injuries among cardiothoracic surgeons is bolstered by a significant lack of institutional support for cardiothoracic surgeons. In a national survey conducted by Mathey-Andrews and colleagues[8], roughly 90% of cardiothoracic surgeons felt that they were not supported by their institution in terms of ergonomics education, assessment, and support. Other studies have echoed this sentiment, all calling on institutions to step up and provide more comprehensive surgical education to their surgeons.[27,51,53] There is a critical need for institutions to take the initiative in prioritizing ergonomic education. This involves not only training, that specifically addresses the unique ergonomic challenges in cardiothoracic surgery, but also institutional policies that encourage the adoption of ergonomic practices, including the provision of ergonomic equipment and regular workshops or training sessions to update surgeons on best practices.

Technological Innovations and Future Directions

The cardiothoracic surgery subspecialty is undergoing transformative changes, and technological innovation could potentially alleviate or worsen ergonomic problems that face cardiothoracic surgeons. For example, robotic surgery, despite being hailed as a technological advance that can lengthen a surgeon's career, is actually associated with increased musculoskeletal pain.[6,8] Other technological innovations that employ the latest advances in artificial intelligence (AI), virtual reality (VR), and wearable technology could potentially reduce ergonomic issues for cardiothoracic surgeons in the future.

Artificial Intelligence in Cardiothoracic Surgery

AI can transform how we perform and teach surgical skills in the OR. Hamilton and colleagues[54] evaluated 13 surgical residents performing simulated laparoscopic tasks before and after reviewing an ergonomics curriculum while being filmed by a sensorless app that uses AI to calculate joint angles. The app then converted these angles to scores based on their deviations from healthy angles.[54] The participants followed up their session by participating in a focus group that discussed surgical ergonomics.[54] Upon completion, residents saw improved neck and shoulder angle ergonomic scores.[54] This study found that AI-based applications could produce promising results to improve ergonomics and ergonomic awareness for surgical residents.[54]

Virtual and Augmented Reality

Virtual reality (VR) and augmented reality (AR) technology offers a safe and effective platform for surgical training, allowing surgeons to practice complex procedures in a simulated environment.[55] This not only enhances the surgeon's skills but also contributes to better ergonomics by allowing them to refine their techniques in a controlled setting.[55] Lim and colleagues[55] evaluated the mental and physical demand exerted on thoracic, laparoscopic, and thyroid surgeons with and without the use of AR glasses that systematically analyzed ergonomic benefits. Surface electromyography (EMG) was used to measure muscle activation and fatigue.[55] The authors found that there was a significant decrease in subjective pain scores as well as a significant decrease in the EMG after using AR glasses.[55] The authors concluded that the AR technology could aid in correcting bad posture in surgeons and reduce overall muscular fatigue in the upper body.[55] Beyond just perioperative applications, VR can be used for preoperative planning, enabling surgeons to visualize and strategize complex surgeries beforehand, potentially leading to more efficient and ergonomic operation techniques.[56]

Wearable Devices and Technology

Wearable technologies are used to monitor and improve the ergonomics of surgeons during operations. Meltzer and colleagues[57] evaluated the impact of using wearable sensor inertial measurement units to assess ergonomic risks. Such devices can be integrated into surgical education to teach residents and medical students better ergonomic techniques to prevent work-related musculoskeletal disorders and ensure career longevity.[57] This technology not only helps in reducing the risk of musculoskeletal injuries but also has the potential to aid in enhancing surgical performance through better ergonomic practices. Piscitelli and colleagues[58] are working on a similar project that evaluates a wearable device that can track bodily posture and tension and provide surgeons with real-time and postoperative feedback.

The data provided from AI, VR/AR, and wearable devices not only have potential to improve the longevity of a CT surgeon's career but could also be used to improve training for future surgeons in medical school and residency.

SUMMARY

In the ever-demanding field of cardiothoracic surgery, optimizing surgical ergonomics is crucial for the health and career of the surgeon. Maintaining static and often uncomfortable positions during long operations leads to musculoskeletal strain and injuries over time. A multifaceted approach to reduce injury includes targeted physical exercises focused on core stability and upper body strength, intraoperative stretching routines, and taking regular microbreaks to alleviate accumulated physical tension. Proper adjustments in table height, monitor placement, and ergonomically designed surgical instruments also play a critical role in minimizing physical strain. Equally important, if an injury occurs, early intervention and comprehensive rehabilitation programs, which include both physical therapy and psychological support, are vital for surgeons experiencing musculoskeletal discomfort. Additionally, there is also a significant need for enhanced surgical ergonomics education and more robust institutional support. Technological innovations, such as AI, VR, and wearable technologies, have the potential to revolutionize surgical ergonomics. Prioritizing surgical ergonomics is critical to wellness and career of cardiothoracic surgeons.

CLINICS CARE POINTS

- Cardiothoracic surgeons are at a significant risk of developing musculoskeletal disorders due to the nature of their surgical procedures.

- There is a tendency among surgeons to postpone seeking medical care for musculoskeletal issues, potentially exacerbating these conditions.

- Implementation of ergonomic practices, including stretching, posture adjustments, and using ergonomically designed surgical instruments, is vital for reducing injury risk.

- Advanced surgical techniques, such as minimally invasive procedures, while beneficial for patients, can pose additional ergonomic challenges for surgeons.

- Institutions should provide adequate support and training in ergonomics to surgeons, emphasizing injury prevention and sustainable practice.

- Embracing technological advancements such as robotic surgery may improve ergonomic conditions but requires proper training and adaptation.

- A combined effort from medical institutions, surgical departments, and individual surgeons is necessary to address and improve ergonomic conditions in cardiothoracic surgery.

DISCLOSURE

The authors have nothing to disclose.

REFERENCES

1. Papaspyros SC, Kar A, O'Regan D. Surgical ergonomics. Analysis of technical skills, simulation models and assessment methods. Int J Surg 2015; 18:83–7.
2. Park A, Lee G, Seagull FJ, et al. Patients benefit while surgeons suffer: an impending epidemic. J Am Coll Surg 2010;210(3):306–13.
3. Voss RK, Chiang YJ, Cromwell KD, et al. Do No Harm, Except to Ourselves? A Survey of Symptoms and Injuries in Oncologic Surgeons and Pilot Study of an Intraoperative Ergonomic Intervention. J Am Coll Surg 2017;224(1):16–25 e1.
4. Seagull FJ. Disparities between industrial and surgical ergonomics. Work 2012;41(Suppl 1):4669–72.
5. Dairywala MI, Gupta S, Salna M, et al. Surgeon Strength: Ergonomics and Strength Training in Cardiothoracic Surgery. Semin Thorac Cardiovasc Surg Winter 2022;34(4):1220–9.
6. Catanzarite T, Tan-Kim J, Whitcomb EL, et al. Ergonomics in Surgery: A Review. Female Pelvic Med Reconstr Surg 2018;24(1):1–12.
7. Epstein S, Sparer EH, Tran BN, et al. Prevalence of Work-Related Musculoskeletal Disorders Among Surgeons and Interventionalists: A Systematic

Review and Meta-analysis. JAMA Surg 2018;153(2): e174947. https://doi.org/10.1001/jamasurg.2017. 4947.

8. Mathey-Andrews CA, Venkateswaran S, McCarthy ML, et al. A national survey of occupational musculoskeletal injuries in cardiothoracic surgeons. J Thorac Cardiovasc Surg 2023. https://doi.org/10.1016/j.jtcvs.2023.08.038.

9. Schlussel AT, Maykel JA. Ergonomics and Musculoskeletal Health of the Surgeon. Clin Colon Rectal Surg 2019;32(6):424–34.

10. Stucky CH, Cromwell KD, Voss RK, et al. Surgeon symptoms, strain, and selections: Systematic review and meta-analysis of surgical ergonomics. Ann Med Surg (Lond). 2018;27:1–8.

11. Cohn LH, Adams DH, Couper GS, et al. Minimally invasive cardiac valve surgery improves patient satisfaction while reducing costs of cardiac valve replacement and repair. Ann Surg 1997;226(4): 421–6 [discussion: 427-8].

12. Iribarne A, Easterwood R, Chan EY, et al. The golden age of minimally invasive cardiothoracic surgery: current and future perspectives. Future Cardiol 2011;7(3):333–46.

13. Soueid A, Oudit D, Thiagarajah S, et al. The pain of surgery: pain experienced by surgeons while operating. Int J Surg 2010;8(2):118–20.

14. Ikonomidis JS, Boden N, Atluri P. The Society of Thoracic Surgeons Thoracic Surgery Practice and Access Task Force-2019 Workforce Report. Ann Thorac Surg 2020;110(3):1082–90.

15. Jensen MJ, Liao J, Van Gorp B, et al. Incorporating Surgical Ergonomics Education into Surgical Residency Curriculum. J Surg Educ 2021;78(4): 1209–15.

16. Aaron KA, Vaughan J, Gupta R, et al. The risk of ergonomic injury across surgical specialties. PLoS One 2021;16(2):e0244868. https://doi.org/10.1371/journal.pone.0244868.

17. Potter AL, Rosenstein AL, Kandala K, et al. Shortage of Thoracic Surgeons in the United States: Implications for Treatment and Survival for Stage I Lung Cancer Patients. J Thorac Cardiovasc Surg 2023. https://doi.org/10.1016/j.jtcvs.2023.08.059.

18. Grover A, Gorman K, Dall TM, et al. Shortage of cardiothoracic surgeons is likely by 2020. Circulation 2009;120(6):488–94.

19. American College of Surgeons Division of Education & Surgical Ergonomics Committee. Surgical Ergonomics Recommendations, *American College of Surgeons Education,* Available at: https://www.facs.org/media/tdeemrnw/23_ed_surgicalergonomics recommendations_pdf_v4.pdf, 2023. Accessed May 23, 2024.

20. Winters JN, Sommer NZ, Romanelli MR, et al. Stretching and Strength Training to Improve Postural Ergonomics and Endurance in the Operating Room.

Plast Reconstr Surg Glob Open 2020;8(5):e2810. https://doi.org/10.1097/GOX.0000000000002810.

21. Kumar T, Kumar S, Nezamuddin M, et al. Efficacy of core muscle strengthening exercise in chronic low back pain patients. J Back Musculoskelet Rehabil 2015;28(4):699–707.

22. Ciolac EG, Rodrigues-da-Silva JM. Resistance Training as a Tool for Preventing and Treating Musculoskeletal Disorders. Sports Med 2016;46(9): 1239–48.

23. Giagio S, Volpe G, Pillastrini P, et al. A Preventive Program for Work-related Musculoskeletal Disorders Among Surgeons: Outcomes of a Randomized Controlled Clinical Trial. Ann Surg 2019;270(6):969–75.

24. Elzomor A, Tunkel A, Lee E, et al. Intraoperative stretching microbreaks reduce surgery-related musculoskeletal pain in otolaryngologists. Am J Otolaryngol 2022;43(6):103594. https://doi.org/10.1016/j.amjoto.2022.103594.

25. Koshy K, Syed H, Luckiewicz A, et al. Interventions to improve ergonomics in the operating theatre: A systematic review of ergonomics training and intraoperative microbreaks. Ann Med Surg (Lond). 2020;55:135–42.

26. Park AE, Zahiri HR, Hallbeck MS, et al. Intraoperative "Micro Breaks" With Targeted Stretching Enhance Surgeon Physical Function and Mental Focus: A Multicenter Cohort Study. Ann Surg 2017; 265(2):340–6.

27. Epstein S, Tran BN, Capone AC, et al. The Current State of Surgical Ergonomics Education in U.S. Surgical Training: A Survey Study. Ann Surg 2019; 269(4):778–84.

28. Matern U, Koneczny S. Safety, hazards and ergonomics in the operating room. Surg Endosc 2007; 21(11):1965–9.

29. Kelts GI, McMains KC, Chen PG, et al. Monitor height ergonomics: A comparison of operating room video display terminals. Allergy Rhinol (Providence) 2015;6(1):28–32.

30. Canadian Centre for Occupational Health and Safety, Working in a Standing Position, *Canadian Centre for Occupational Health and Safety,* Accessed May 23, 2024, Available at: https://www.ccohs.ca/oshanswers/ergonomics/standing/standing_basic.html, 2023.

31. Moore SM, Torma-Krajewski, J., Steiner, L. J., Practical Demonstrations of Ergonomic Principles, *National Institute for Occupational Safety and Health,* Accessed May 23, 2024, Available at: https://www.cdc.gov/niosh/media/pdfs/2011-191_demonsttaion-of-ergonomic-principles.pdf, 2011.

32. Unver S, Makal Organ E. The effect of anti-fatigue floor mat on pain and fatigue levels of surgical team members: A crossover study. Appl Ergon 2023;110:104017. https://doi.org/10.1016/j.apergo.2023.104017.

33. Aghazadeh J, Ghaderi M, Azghani MR, et al. Anti-fatigue mats, low back pain, and electromyography: An interventional study. Int J Occup Med Environ Health 2015;28(2):347–56.

34. Koseki T, Kakizaki F, Hayashi S, et al. Effect of forward head posture on thoracic shape and respiratory function. J Phys Ther Sci 2019;31(1):63–8.

35. Ciancaglini R, Testa M, Radaelli G. Association of neck pain with symptoms of temporomandibular dysfunction in the general adult population. Scand J Rehabil Med 1999;31(1):17–22.

36. Lee WY, Okeson JP, Lindroth J. The relationship between forward head posture and temporomandibular disorders. J Orofac Pain. Spring 1995;9(2):161–7.

37. Szeto GP, Straker L, Raine S. A field comparison of neck and shoulder postures in symptomatic and asymptomatic office workers. Appl Ergon 2002; 33(1):75–84.

38. Fernandez-de-las-Penas C, Alonso-Blanco C, Cuadrado ML, et al. Forward head posture and neck mobility in chronic tension-type headache: a blinded, controlled study. Cephalalgia 2006;26(3): 314–9.

39. Walker B., Duke surgery introduces ergonomics program to improve surgeon health. Duke surgery, Duke University School of Medicine, Available at: https://surgery.duke.edu/news/duke-surgery-introduces-ergonomics-program-improve-surgeon-health, 2017. Accessed May 23, 2024.

40. Kaplan DJ, Patel JN, Liporace FA, et al. Intraoperative radiation safety in orthopaedics: a review of the ALARA (As low as reasonably achievable) principle. Patient Saf Surg 2016;10:27.

41. Scheidt S, Ossendorf R, Prangenberg C, et al. The Impact of Lead Aprons on Posture of Orthopaedic Surgeons. Z für Orthop Unfallchirurgie 2022; 160(1):56–63. Der Einfluss von Rontgenschurzen auf die Korperhaltung von Orthopaden und Unfallchirurgen.

42. Supe AN, Kulkarni GV, Supe PA. Ergonomics in laparoscopic surgery. J Minimal Access Surg 2010;6(2):31–6.

43. Nordeman L, Nilsson B, Moller M, et al. Early access to physical therapy treatment for subacute low back pain in primary health care: a prospective randomized clinical trial. Clin J Pain 2006;22(6): 505–11.

44. Zigenfus GC, Yin J, Giang GM, et al. Effectiveness of early physical therapy in the treatment of acute low back musculoskeletal disorders. J Occup Environ Med 2000;42(1):35–9.

45. Swinkels IC, van den Ende CH, van den Bosch W, et al. Physiotherapy management of low back pain: does practice match the Dutch guidelines? Aust J Physiother 2005;51(1):35–41.

46. Gellhorn AC, Chan L, Martin B, et al. Management patterns in acute low back pain: the role of physical therapy. Spine 2012;37(9):775–82.

47. El-Tallawy SN, Nalamasu R, Salem GI, et al. Management of Musculoskeletal Pain: An Update with Emphasis on Chronic Musculoskeletal Pain. Pain Ther 2021;10(1):181–209.

48. Gennarelli SM, Brown SM, Mulcahey MK. Psychosocial interventions help facilitate recovery following musculoskeletal sports injuries: a systematic review. Phys Sportsmed 2020;48(4):370–7.

49. Verrier ED. The Elite Athlete, the Master Surgeon. J Am Coll Surg 2017;224(3):225–35.

50. Ponzer S, Molin U, Johansson SE, et al. Psychosocial support in rehabilitation after orthopedic injuries. J Trauma 2000;48(2):273–9.

51. Pierce SM, Heiman AJ, Ricci JA. Evaluating the Current State of Ergonomics Education Offered to Students in US Medical Students. Am Surg 2023; 89(5):1798–806.

52. Sergesketter AR, Lubkin DT, Shammas RL, et al. The Impact of Ergonomics on Recruitment to Surgical Fields: A Multi-Institutional Survey Study. J Surg Res 2019;236:238–46.

53. Buddle V, Nugent R, Jack RA 2nd, et al. Orthopedists Report High Prevalence of Work-Related Pain and Low Ergonomic Awareness. Orthopedics 2023;46(5):280–4.

54. Hamilton BC, Dairywala MI, Highet A, et al. Artificial intelligence based real-time video ergonomic assessment and training improves resident ergonomics. Am J Surg 2023;226(5):741–6.

55. Lim AK, Ryu J, Yoon HM, et al. Ergonomic effects of medical augmented reality glasses in video-assisted surgery. Surg Endosc 2022;36(2):988–98.

56. Louis RG, Steinberg GK, Duma C, et al. Early Experience With Virtual and Synchronized Augmented Reality Platform for Preoperative Planning and Intraoperative Navigation: A Case Series. Oper Neurosurg (Hagerstown) 2021;21(4):189–96.

57. Meltzer AJ, Hallbeck MS, Morrow MM, et al. Measuring Ergonomic Risk in Operating Surgeons by Using Wearable Technology. JAMA Surg 2020; 155(5):444–6.

58. Piscitelli G, Anderson T, Buban P, et al. Wearable devices to track body's posture and tension. 2023. Accessed May 23, 2024, Available at: https://bmedesign.engr.wisc.edu/projects/f23/ergonomic_sensing.

Wellness Strategies Among Bad Outcomes and Complications

Ian C. Bostock, MD, MS[a],*, Mara B. Antonoff, MD[b]

KEYWORDS

- Wellness • Bad outcomes • Postoperative complications • Litigation • Lawsuits
- Transition into practice

KEY POINTS

- "Second victims" refer to health care providers who have been involved in unanticipated adverse events, medical errors, or patient-related injuries, and subsequently become traumatized by the event.
- Patient care is a team sport. The traditional view of having the surgeon be the sole responsible individual for the patient's outcome is honorable, but an outdated concept.
- Doctors experiencing untoward consequences of medical errors may develop heightened self-doubt, greater insecurity, and imposter syndrome.
- Our primary commitment as doctors is to take care of our patients. This objective is the upmost priority for all clinicians, and surgeons are not the exception.
- Acquiring a growth mindset in surgery, is a critical aspect of maturing as a clinician and avoiding or adapting to the emotional, intellectual, and physical toll in this profession.

BACKGROUND: BAD OUTCOMES IN CARDIOTHORACIC SURGERY

> In thoracic surgery, the surgeon is dealing with vital functions. It is quite apparent that in this field, far more than in any other surgical field, his major considerations, and efforts must be directed toward prevention of complications or at least their recognition and prompt treatment. Otherwise, these operations will be attended by many serious complications.
>
> —Herbert Adams and David Boyd.[1]

As cardiothoracic surgeons, the authors perform complex interventions on patients with serious comorbidities, requiring multidisciplinary collaboration and often flawless conduct of extensive operations.[2] There are numerous opportunities for undesired outcomes, even in the presence of comprehensive and conscientious care throughout all preoperative planning, intraoperative decision-making, and postoperative management. Surgery of the chest is high stakes, and adverse events are common.

Second Victims

Given the frequency and severity of such complications, cardiothoracic surgeons are at particularly high risk of becoming *second victims*.[3] "Second victims" refer to physicians and other health care providers who have been involved in unanticipated adverse events, medical errors, or patient-related injuries, and subsequently become traumatized by the event.[4] It has been estimated

[a] Department of Cardiothoracic Surgery, Medical University of South Carolina, 30 Courtenay Drive, Charleston, SC 29425, USA; [b] Division of Surgery, Department of Thoracic and Cardiovascular Surgery, University of Texas MD Anderson Cancer Center, 1400 Pressler Street Unit 1489, Houston, TX 77030, USA
* Corresponding author.
E-mail address: bostock.ian@gmail.com

Thorac Surg Clin 34 (2024) 207–212
https://doi.org/10.1016/j.thorsurg.2024.04.009
1547-4127/24/© 2024 Elsevier Inc. All rights reserved.

that 30% to 40% of healthcare workers who are involved in such circumstances go on to experience harmful personal impact,[5] and this may be particularly prevalent among cardiothoracic surgeons, who tend to take on the roles of team leaders, decision makers, and primary procedural technicians. In one series, 83% of physicians reported involvement in adverse events, with more than 3-quarters acknowledging subsequent downstream effects to their personal and professional lives.[6] It's important to recognize that certain populations of surgeons in our workforce may be particularly susceptible to second-victim phenomena, and these tend to be those individuals who are demographically underrepresented, already often feeling like their performances are magnified, inspected to a greater extent than their peers, while feeling a sense of isolationism.[3] Several authors have shown that women are likely more intrinsically prone than men to develop emotional sequelae of medical errors,[7,8] and given their persistently low numbers in our field, these issues may be further amplified among women cardiothoracic surgeons. Our trainees, including residents and fellows are also more likely to be at risk of personalization and traumatic sequelae of the mistakes that inevitably occur on the front lines of complex patient care.[3]

The manifestations of second-victim phenomena vary widely, and they can be quite damaging. Traumatized surgeons may develop symptoms including anxiety, depression, fear, guilt, and shame.[3] Some individuals may develop somatic symptoms or even posttraumatic stress disorder.[9] Moreover, emotions of self-loathing and self-deprecation, as well as helplessness in the overall situation, can lead to substance abuse, addiction, self-harm, and suicidal ideation or actions.[10] Individuals may behave differently around loved ones, impacting their relationships—the very relationships and support that may have otherwise been helpful in navigating the stress surrounding the situation. Consequences may include strained relationships, estrangement, and divorce. Previous investigators have demonstrated that involvement in patient complications has led physicians to report more frequent burnout, greater level of exhaustion, and overall lower quality of life.[11]

Not only do these circumstances harm the health care provider but also they also harm our patients. Doctors experiencing untoward consequences of medical errors may develop heightened self-doubt, greater insecurity, and imposter syndrome—and they may be reluctant to address future near misses or admit errors.[3] As such, this could directly result in delayed recognition and management of other complications along with failure to fix systematic problems.

RISING FROM THE ASHES: STRATEGIES FOR COPING, SURVIVING, AND THRIVING
First, Take Care of the Patient

The authors' primary commitment as doctors is to take care of our patients. This objective is the upmost priority for all clinicians, and surgeons are not the exception. When a treatment or procedure that the authors provide fails or there are serious downstream adverse events, they believe like they have betrayed their patient and this primary commitment. This feeling of failure or guilt can lead us to shy away from continuing to care for that patient.

An important distinction must be made between adverse events resulting in morbidity versus mortality; when a patient experiences an untoward outcome less than death, thorough and conscientious efforts must be put toward optimizing that patient's outcome going forward. As stated by Dr Kraev and Perez-Tamayo, "A thousand things must go right for a patient to do well. Every case is another opportunity to perfect another one of those thousand details".[12]

It is at this precise moment, when the clinician should realize that the patients are at their most vulnerable and needs us more than ever. The authors' have to ensure that the patients are being taken care of in the most comprehensive way. It is ok if the primary provider of medical care changes while the surgeon takes a step back and evaluates how they are feeling (ie, involving a partner or colleague), but he or she should never abandon the patient. The physician-patient relationship should continue throughout this entire event. Achieving and maintaining patient safety must absolutely be prioritized. This often means bringing on additional resources and team members, which should be undertaken without hesitation and with an abundance of humility. The authors aim to do no harm, and, if they find ourselves in a situation where harm has been done, they must work diligently to provide safety and healing.

Next, Heal Thyself: Managing Emotions

When a clinician is faced with a difficult patient situation or a negative outcome after an unsuccessful procedure, he or she is also confronted with a myriad of emotions that can make recovery or processing of this event quite challenging. There has been a lot of work trying to establish a best practice of processing these events and help clinicians heal.[13–15] The authors have found the work of best-selling author Dr Brene Brown to be quite interesting and applicable to the struggles they face. Dr Brown has focused a significant amount of her career in investigating the relationship between guilt and shame. In her research, Dr Brown states that shame is part of the human experience regardless of the exposure to trauma. The authors tend to avoid feeling shame because it leaves us feeling vulnerable and uncomfortable but if they don't face shame head on, it ends up spreading fear, and encouraging negative behavior, negative thinking, and burnout.[16]

Dr Brown defines shame as the intensely painful feeling or experience of believing that the authors are flawed and therefore unworthy of love, belonging, and connection. She further explains that shame consists of 3 pillars: it is universal, it is difficult to discuss, and talking about shame helps us overcome it and build a stronger sense of self. The authors are all capable of overcoming shame by building what Brown describes as "shame resilience" which consists of having (1) capacity to recognize when they are experiencing shame and asking for what they need, (2) ability to move through the feeling of shame with authenticity and growth, and (3) building connections and empathy with people around you. In essence, dealing with shame is not black or white; it is a continuum between shame (fear, blame, and disconnection) and empathy (courage, compassion, and connection).[16]

In her book, Daring Greatly, Dr Brown highlights the importance of empathy and vulnerability as the ultimate antidote to shame. Vulnerability is the cornerstone of courage, resilience, and problem solving. Connection is a vital aspect of shame resilience, enabling them to believe valued, affirmed, and accepted. She recommends practicing self-kindness over self-judgement, practicing common humanity over isolation, and mindfulness rather than over-identification.[16]

After a poor surgical outcome, a mistake, or an adverse event, the initial human response may be to withdraw or avoid contact with the patient or their family. Even though this human response is understandable and natural, it may have the undesired effect of disturbing the patient-physician relationship, human connection, and eventually lead to feelings of anger, resentment, or misunderstanding in the patient, their family, and the physician.[13–15] As mentioned earlier, when dealing with a situation that brings us shame, the authors should seek human connection, empathy, and vulnerability. Showing up with an open mind, open heart, and full honesty is the most powerful way to show the patient the power of their physician's commitment to their care. Mistakes happen and will continue to happen, but the way the authors deal with

them is of the outmost importance. Several authors have documented the importance of maintaining an honest relationship with the patient and their family through a bad outcome, with some studies even showing the protective effect of communication and avoiding lawsuits.[17]

Patient care is a team sport. The traditional view of having the surgeon be the sole responsible individual for the patient's outcome is honorable, but in the authors' opinion, an outdated concept. A single person cannot be responsible for every single detail of patient care and even though surgical culture has motivated us to assume full responsibility, patients are taken care in a systematic fashion with multiple individuals providing valuable contributions to the outcome. The importance of including multiple clinical teams, nursing staff, physical therapists, social workers, and so forth to the patient care team cannot be understated. When dealing with a poor outcome, having the input from multiple teams may prove invaluable and may help with the patient and their family feel more supported and given an improved sense of transparency.[13–15,18,19] Using clear language with a unified message among the care teams will help solidify the connection with the patients and their family and lead to an improved patient-physician relationship.[13–15,18,19]

It has been shown by numerous authors that debriefing activities may reduce physician burnout through enhancement of social support and interprofessional collaboration.[20–24] As with many other challenges in medicine, it is clear that preventing burnout is more effective than trying to fix established burnout,[18] and employing timely and proactive debriefing may serve this end. There are several strategies for debriefing, with one described approach utilizing "Death Cafes," which include a specific structured form. These event the aim to foster reflection on distressing patient events while developing a sense of community and collaboration among members of the team.[25] Thus, one of the important steps of taking care of *oneself* emphasizes the community support of networking—which ties in closely with the simultaneous need to take care of the *other* members of the team.

Taking Care of Your Team

While surgeons often tend to focus their efforts after a complication on dealing with the patient and family members, it is critically important for the surgeon to recognize that there are numerous additional team members who may be struggling with the negative impact of the event. The multidisciplinary team composition will vary based on the location of the event, whether it is in the operating room, intensive care unit, surgical ward, or the ambulatory clinic. In all of these settings, there may be nurses, advanced care practitioners, trainees, surgical technologists, anesthesiologists, and many other multidisciplinary team members present—and they all look to the surgeon as the *de facto* team leader. This should be considered an opportunity to bring the team together, to grow as a group, and to strengthen the team's effectiveness, safety, and social bonds.

D'Angelo and colleagues gathered input from operating room team personnel on positive and negative coping strategies of surgeons following adverse intraoperative events. Several themes emerged as being appreciated and valued by team members[15]: (1) they pause or remain calm, (2) they take actions to enhance team cohesion, (3) they obtain help if necessary, (4) they develop and convey a plan, (5) they continue forward fix the problem, and (6) they take responsibility. These approaches are likely to enable the team to grow together. When specifically aiming to enhance team cohesion, specific actions including formal debriefing, informal "checking in" on team members, and providing meaningful appreciation for the value that others have brought to the challenging situation can be particularly helpful.

D'Angelo also identified themes in terms of surgeon behaviors that were not helpful for the team.[15] These included: (1) creating a stressful environment through displays of panic or anxiety, (2) reverting to aggressive or discourteous behavior, resulting in animosity and discord, (3) failing to obtain help when necessary, (4) doesn't have or articulate a clear plan, (5) taking ineffective actions, and (6) blaming others or failing to take responsibility.

Positive and improved team dynamics may emerge from crisis if the team works together to cope. Much of this culture and direction can originate from the attitudes and goals of the surgeon. As surgeons, the authors have the opportunity to bring our teams together after such events, and they should acknowledge and step up to this role.

Managing the Administrative and Legal Needs

Cardiothoracic surgery is among the leading specialties to face malpractice lawsuits, with almost 20% of cardiothoracic surgeons facing some type of lawsuit over a period of 15 years of practice. Additionally, today's environment has brought a physician-patient relationship that differs from historical culture. Practicing medicine has become more structured and formal, and doctors are no longer regarded as infallible and beyond questioning. Corporatization of health care has made it like any other business, and the medical profession is increasingly being guided by motives of profit rather than those of service. Simultaneously, a well-publicized malpractice case can ruin the doctor's career and practice.[26]

Common sense would guide to the fact that the best way to handle medico-legal issues is by preventing them. However, despite all efforts to minimize frequency, such events are impossible to eliminate altogether. Raveesh and colleagues have previously highlighted key preventive measures in safeguarding the doctor against a negligence suit (listed in **Fig. 1**) following an adverse

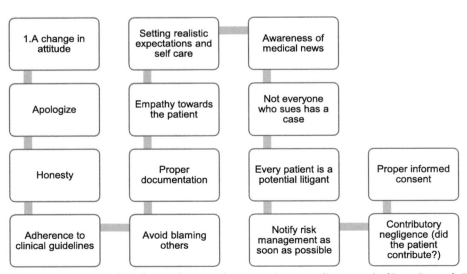

Fig. 1. Key preventive measures in safeguarding the doctor against a negligence suit. (*From* Raveesh BN, Nayak RB, Kumbar SF. Preventing medico-legal issues in clinical practice. Ann Indian Acad Neurol. 2016 Oct;19(Suppl 1):S15-S20. https://doi.org/10.4103/0972-2327.192886. PMID: 27891020; PMCID: PMC5109754.)

event.[26] Through their discussion, the authors emphasize that it is clear that a strong sense of empathy, honesty, clear, and frequent communication, and thorough documentation will protect the physician from a harmful lawsuit. Involving key players in the hospital environment such as partners, colleagues, nursing staff, and risk management, among others, can help protect the physician and highlight the efforts from everyone involved in patient care.

NOW WHAT: GROWING FOR THE FUTURE

Mindset theory holds that those who possess a growth mindset are open to learning from opportunities. They welcome challenges, show a willingness to persist, view effort as tied to mastery, learn from criticism, and view the success of others as a learning moment. It is postulated that these traits allow those with a growth mindset to continue achieving throughout their careers.[27]

The authors think that acquiring a growth mindset in surgery, is a critical aspect of maturing as a clinician and avoiding or adapting to the emotional, intellectual, and physical toll this profession has on surgeons as individuals. Taking time to reflect on one's accomplishments and failures through a lens that highlights what went well and what can be better, can help provide perspective, and strategies to move toward the next case and the next patient more successfully. Additionally, meditation, self-care (such as exercise, balanced diet, or social interactions), journaling, breathing techniques, counseling, and professional coaching can be powerful tools to help surgeons avoid burnout and thrive in the art of surgery. Specific interventions such as thorough assessment of morbidity and mortality events with other colleagues, root cause analysis, and systematic changes to prevent future complications are key steps for growing after these events.

DISCLOSURE

The authors have nothing to disclosures.

REFERENCES

1. Adams HD, Boyd DP. Complications of thoracic surgery. Surg Clin 1957;37(3):615–24.
2. Martinez EA, Thompson DA, Errett NA, et al. High stakes and high risk: a focused qualitative review of hazards during cardiac surgery. Anesth Analg 2011;112(5):1061–74.
3. Chen S, Skidmore S, Ferrigno BN, et al. The second victim of unanticipated adverse events. J Thorac Cardiovasc Surg 2023;166(3):890–4.
4. Scott SD, Hirschinger LE, Cox KR, et al. The natural history of recovery for the healthcare provider "second victim" after adverse patient events. BMJ Qual Saf 2009;18(5):325–30.
5. Seys D, Wu AW, Gerven EV, et al. Health care professionals as second victims after adverse events: a systematic review. Eval Health Prof 2013;36(2):135–62.
6. Harrison R, Lawton R, Stewart K. Doctors' experiences of adverse events in secondary care: the professional and personal impact. Clin Med 2014;14(6):585.
7. Waterman AD, Garbutt J, Hazel E, et al. The emotional impact of medical errors on practicing physicians in the United States and Canada. Joint Comm J Qual Patient Saf 2007;33(8):467–76.
8. Khansa I, Pearson GD. Coping and recovery in surgical residents after adverse events: the second victim phenomenon. Plastic and Reconstructive Surgery Global Open 2022;10(3):e4203.
9. Coughlan B, Powell D, Higgins MF. The second victim: a review. Eur J Obstet Gynecol Reprod Biol 2017;213:11–6.
10. Christensen JF, Levinson W, Dunn PM. The heart of darkness: the impact of perceived mistakes on physicians. J Gen Intern Med 1992;7:424–31.
11. West CP, Huschka MM, Novotny PJ, et al. Association of perceived medical errors with resident distress and empathy: a prospective longitudinal study. JAMA 2006;296(9):1071–8.
12. Kraev AI, Perez-Tamayo RA. A Gnostic Understanding of Coping for the Cardiothoracic Surgeon. Tex Heart Inst J 2022;49(4):e217657.
13. Anton NE, Montero PN, Howley LD, et al. What stress coping strategies are surgeons relying upon during surgery? Am J Surg 2015;210(5):846–51.
14. D'Angelo JD, Lund S, Busch RA, et al. Coping with errors in the operating room: Intraoperative strategies, postoperative strategies, and sex differences. Surgery 2021;170(2):440–5.
15. D'Angelo ALD, Kapur N, Kelley SR, et al. The good, the bad, and the ugly: Operative staff perspectives of surgeon coping with intraoperative errors. Surgery 2023;174(2):222–8.
16. Brown B. Daring greatly: how the courage to be vulnerable transforms the way we live, love, parent, and lead. London: Penguin; 2015.
17. Watrelot AA, Tanos V, Grimbizis G, et al. From complication to litigation: The importance of non-technical skills in the management of complications. Facts, Views & Vision in ObGyn 2020;12(2):133.
18. Sinskey JL, Margolis RD, Vinson AE. The wicked problem of physician well-being. Anesthesiol Clin 2022;40(2):213–23.
19. Liukka M, Steven A, Vizcaya Moreno MF, et al. Action after adverse events in healthcare: an integrative

literature review. Int J Environ Res Publ Health 2020; 17(13):4717.

20. Govindan M, Keefer P, Sturza J, et al. Empowering residents to process distressing events: a debriefing workshop. MedEdPORTAL 2019;15:10809.

21. Eagle S, Creel A, Alexandrov A. The effect of facilitated peer support sessions on burnout and grief management among health care providers in pediatric intensive care units: a pilot study. J Palliat Med 2012;15(11):1178–80.

22. Browning ED, Cruz JS. Reflective debriefing: a social work intervention addressing moral distress among ICU nurses. J Soc Work End-of-Life Palliat Care 2018;14(1):44–72.

23. Abrams MP. Improving resident well-being and burnout: the role of peer support. Journal of Graduate Medical Education 2017;9(2):264.

24. Ziegelstein RC. Creating structured opportunities for social engagement to promote well-being and avoid burnout in medical students and residents. Acad Med 2018;93(4):537–9.

25. Hammer R, Ravindran N, Nielsen N. Can Death Cafés resuscitate morale in hospitals? Med Humanit 2021;47(1):2–3.

26. Raveesh BN, Nayak RB, Kumbar SF. Preventing medico-legal issues in clinical practice. Ann Indian Acad Neurol 2016 Oct;19(Suppl 1):S15–20.

27. Dweck CS. Mindset: the new psychology of success. New York: Random House; 2006.

Sleep, Nutrition, and Health Maintenance in Cardiothoracic Surgery

Joseph M. Obeid, MD[a], John K. Sadeghi, MD[a], Andrea S. Wolf, MD, MPH[b], Ross M. Bremner, MD, PhD[c,d],*

KEYWORDS

- Cardiothoracic surgeons • Well-being • Wellness • Sleep • Nutrition • Health • Exercise • Self-care

KEY POINTS

- Cardiothoracic (CT) surgeons should aim to maintain well-being.
- Maintaining well-being will help prolong a CT surgeon's career and will set one up to provide the best patient care.
- CT surgeons can maintain well-being through adequate sleep, proper nutrition, regular exercise, and routine health maintenance.

INTRODUCTION

Physician burnout is at an all-time high. While there is significant attention being paid to the causes and solutions, many of which may be institutional responsibilities, this article deals with some basic health needs over which each cardiothoracic (CT) surgeon has some control. Paying attention to these basics is essential for overall physician well-being. CT surgeons are subjected to prolonged work hours and particularly stressful conditions. These factors impact the ability of the surgeon to prioritize the basic needs of sleep, nutrition, and health maintenance (such as exercise). This article discusses the importance of these basic needs and will present possible strategies to help us prioritize them in our day-to-day lives.

CT surgeons are in some ways unique. The magnitude and duration of many operations are often "life or death" situations, creating significant stress on the physician. Outcomes are not always perfect although we continually strive to make them so. Many of these operations are emergent and as such are very disruptive to the regular routine of the surgeon. A busy day trying to manage an operative or clinic schedule can be interrupted by a transplant or an aortic dissection, for example, and many of these urgent operations are done after normal hours, again disrupting possible plans for a trip to the gym, a healthy dinner, and a good night's sleep.

We will discuss how important sleep, nutrition, and exercise are, how we have historically sacrificed these in our mission to always put the patient first, and how prioritizing these has the potential to improve not only the health of the CT surgeon, but also the outcomes of their operations, their relationships with their colleagues and their own families, and their overall sense of well-being.

Our gladiator culture (think: "The problem with every other night call is that you miss half the

[a] Department of Cardiothoracic Surgery, Temple University Hospital, 3401 N Broad Street, Parkinson Pavilion, Suite 501C, Philadelphia, PA 19140, USA; [b] New York Mesothelioma Program, Department of Thoracic Surgery, The Icahn School of Medicine at Mount Sinai, 1190 Fifth Avenue, Box 1023, New York, NY 10029, USA; [c] Norton Thoracic Institute, St. Joseph's Hospital and Medical Center, 500 W. Thomas Road, Suite 500, Phoenix, AZ 85013, USA; [d] School of Medicine, Creighton University, Phoenix Health Sciences Campus, 3100 N Central Avenue, Phoenix, AZ 85012, USA
* Corresponding author.
E-mail address: ross.bremner@dignityhealth.org

Thorac Surg Clin 34 (2024) 213–221
https://doi.org/10.1016/j.thorsurg.2024.04.004

good cases" or "To ask for help is weakness"), while proving our resilience to long-term stress and fatigue, has now been shown to have many negative effects. It is time we paid attention to our health so that we can bring our best selves to the needs of our patients and to those we care most about.

SLEEP

Sleep: "You can sleep when you die"—the adage that was talked about during many of our residencies. In his TED talk "Sleep is your Superpower," Matthew Walker covers the importance of sleep in our lives, and how detrimental poor or decreased sleep can be, from impaired immunity[1] to decreased testicle size! Sleep deprivation increases the risk of hypertension[2] and cardiometabolic diseases[3] as well as many negative impacts on both physical and mental health.

Quality of Sleep

Five stages of sleep characterize a cycle of sleep which variably lasts, in adults, from 70 to 100 minutes in the first cycle and 90 to 120 minutes in subsequent sleep cycles. These can be monitored and identified on polysomnogram studies. Stages are categorized as rapid eye movement (REM) sleep or deep sleep (comprising 20%–25% of each cycle), and 4 non-REM (NREM) sleep stages (comprising 75%–80% of the cycle).[4] NREM is essential for learning and building memory[5] as well as motor skills, including speed and accuracy,[6] qualities required to perform surgery. Increased NREM sleep was significantly associated with improved performance overnight of motor skill tasks.[7] REM stage is characterized by low-amplitude high-frequency activity on polysomnogram accompanied by REM and muscle fasciculations.[8] It is also termed "active sleep" due to high-frequency electroencephalogram (EEG) activity similar to that of awake EEG coupled with active suppression of skeletal muscles.[9] The amount of total REM sleep is critical for sleep quality[10] and is essential for a sense of well-being and for an individual's creativity.[11] Dreaming occurs during REM sleep when muscle tone is lost to avoid enacting dreams. Twitching that occurs during REM sleep is believed to contribute to the development of the sensorimotor system by stimulating certain individual muscles against a silent background.[12,13] REM lasts 1 to 5 minutes in the first sleep cycle and is progressively longer in subsequent sleep cycles.[4] As a result, most REM sleep occurs in the latter half of the night and is severely decreased by interrupted sleeping.[10] Similarly, decreasing total time asleep by only 10% results in a disproportionate loss of

REM sleep (perhaps >20%). A total of 1.5 to 2 hours of total REM sleep is needed for a healthy night's sleep.[4] This underlines the importance of uninterrupted sleep to obtain adequate amounts of total REM sleep. Interrupting sleep even if only for a few minutes to answer a call can disrupt these cycles and significantly reduce overall REM sleep. Furthermore, decision-making after abruptly interrupted sleep can be impaired ("fuzzing thinking").[11] After a night of sleep deprivation, the body will prioritize NREM sleep over REM sleep the following night during "sleep rebound."[11] Interrupted sleep night after night, which is often the norm for a CT surgeon, can profoundly deprive surgeons of proper sleep, impacting their well-being, relationships, ability to handle stress, and clinical decisions for their patients (**Fig. 1**).

Sleep assessment tools are useful for self and peer evaluation of sleep habits. They are readily available online and include the Pittsburg Sleep Quality Index, Sleep Quality Scale, Epworth Sleepiness Scale, and Multiple Sleep Latency Test. These tests are summarized in (**Table 1**) and are worth using to evaluate the quality of your own sleep.

Quantity of Sleep

There is a misconception among surgeons that sleep duration is not that important, that we can survive on 4 or 5 hours of sleep each night and still perform optimally. The recommended daily duration of sleep for most adults, however, is at least 7 hours. Sleeping 6 hours or less per night for 14 consecutive days causes cognitive deficits comparable to those of complete sleep deprivation (ie, no sleep at all) for 2 consecutive nights.[14] After 17 to 19 hours without sleep, performance on cognitive tests and response speeds are reduced, mimicking the effect of alcohol intoxication with blood alcohol levels of 0.05% (driving under the influence laws are enforced for individuals with levels 0.04% and higher). With longer periods of

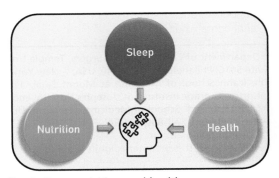

Fig. 1. Sleep, nutrition, and health.

Table 1
Sleep scales and tests

Test/Scale	Factors Included	Outcome
Pittsburg Sleep Quality Index	Hours of sleep, subjective sleep quality, sleep latency, sleep duration, habitual sleep efficiency, sleep disturbances, use of sleeping medication, and daytime dysfunction	Sleep disturbances
Sleep Quality Scale	Daytime symptoms, restoration after sleep, problems initiating and maintaining sleep, difficulty waking, and sleep satisfaction	Quality of sleep
Epworth Sleepiness Scale	Chance of dozing	Daytime sleepiness
Multiple Sleep Latency Test	Takes place the day after an overnight without sleep, under polysomnography evaluation	Quality of sleep

sleep deprivation, impairment reached levels observed with blood alcohol levels of 0.1%.[15] One experiment compared experienced gynecologists performing laparoscopic skills while intoxicated at greater than 0.08% blood alcohol level to those who were sleep deprived with less than 3 hours of sleep in 24 hours. Investigators found that performance was equal between the two groups.[16] Surgeons would like to think they are more trained and ready for sleep deprivation than people in other professions; however, sleep deprivation has been found to negatively impact surgical dexterity.[17] Moreover, surgical trainees have been examined doing simulated tasks on mornings after regular sleep, after a night of decreased sleep, and after a night of no sleep. These studies found that decreased sleep significantly increased stress, errors, and time to complete tasks in a linear manner.[18] Psychological stress, in turn, was associated with increased amplitude of hand tremors shown by an electrophysiology study.[19] Sleep deprivation experiments in an experienced microsurgeon confirmed the declining quality of anastomoses made after sleep deprivation due to a noticeable decline in the surgeon's visuospatial abilities.[20] The effect of sleep deprivation is still somewhat contentious, and more research is needed. Some studies have found little decline in performance of routine surgical tasks performed after sleep deprivation.[21–23] One study testing chronic fatigue over 7 days of sleep deprivation found that tasks were most impaired after the first night of sleep deprivation with relative improvement in the subsequent days, possibly due to adaptation to chronic fatigue.[24] Surgical tasks aside, sleep deprivation of surgeons had a greater negative effect on tasks with higher cognitive demands than those with lower cognitive demand.[25] Knowing this may help tailor post-call requirements to minimal tasks, if necessary.

There is a misconception that one can easily catch up on sleep and that sleep deprivation can easily be reversed. One study revealed that surgeons' sleep patterns were most affected by acute and chronic sleep deprivation on post-call day 2 and that sleep patterns did not return to baseline until day 3.[26] With high-stress situations, complex cases, and prolonged call shifts, CT surgeons are at risk of succumbing to the effects of sleep deprivation without frequent chances to recover. A more recent study has shown that lung transplants done in the daytime have better outcomes than those done at night, likely reflecting the effects of sleep deprivation on all team members.[27] System-based approaches to ensure that CT surgeons sleep appropriately and have time for recovery after losing sleep are critical to CT surgeons' well-being—and likely to the outcomes of our patients.

Effect of Substances on Sleep

Caffeine is a psychoactive substance often used to avoid daytime sleepiness and increase morning arousal. Eighty-five percent of the US population consumes one or more caffeinated beverages per day.[28] Coffee is usually readily available in most hospitals, and intake is very common by most health care workers. Several studies have shown that increasing doses of caffeine are associated with worsening quality of sleep quantified by sleep latency, sleep efficiency, and wake time after sleep onset,[29] to the point that coffee consumption in the evening may be used to induce symptoms and polysomnography tracings mimicking insomnia.[30] A common misconception among high-intensity workers is that the use of coffee counteracts sleep deprivation. While it is true that caffeine as an adenosine receptor antagonist does increase wakefulness and can improve performance, it is doubtful that it can counter all the negative effects of sleep deprivation. In one study, novice surgical trainees were subjected to sleep deprivation and then administered caffeine and taurine: caffeine and taurine were found to restore reaction time and decrease subjective sleepiness but were not found to decrease mistakes.[31] Caffeine intake was also associated with a detrimental effect on novice microsurgeon skills.[32] Clearly, minimizing caffeine intake and avoiding caffeine late in the day will allow for better quality of sleep and subsequently improved well-being. Caffeine has a variable half-life of 2 to 10 hours and when taken later in the day has a significant impact on the quality of sleep in many individuals.[33] Caffeine withdrawal also has negative impacts on performance.[33]

Alcohol is one of the most used "over-the-counter" sleep aids.[34] It has also been cited as a legal compound that is used by health care workers to self-medicate under stress. A recent survey of 1000 health care workers showed that 21% of health care workers consume alcohol or controlled substances multiple times a day.[35] Oreskovich and colleagues[36] found that alcohol abuse or dependence was 13.9% for male surgeons and 25.6% for female surgeons. While alcohol may have multiple negative effects on health and performance, our discussion here is confined to its effects on sleep. Although alcohol may help with falling asleep, it has been shown to impair sleep quality in many ways, and it may affect occasional alcohol users differently than habitual users or alcoholics. Those with alcohol-use disorder have sleep disruptions characterized by insomnia, daytime sleepiness, and altered sleep.[37] Dependence on alcohol to fall asleep follows. When these individuals abstain from alcohol, they experience withdrawal which will induce further insomnia[34] (**Fig. 2**).

Benzodiazepines are commonly prescribed to treat insomnia. This class of drugs may reduce sleep fragmentation and increase NREM sleep, giving the subjective feeling of improved sleep. However, it disrupts other sleep cycles and decreases REM sleep.[38] Benzodiazepines also exacerbate respiratory sleep disorders such as sleep apnea in heavy snorers.[39] Benzodiazepines are very addictive and can induce poor and risky decision-making, so clearly they should never be taken when a surgeon is on call.[40]

Over-the-counter sleep aids such as doxylamine and other antihistamines such as Benadryl (often present in nighttime cold remedies) also affect quality of sleep and may lead to drowsiness and irritability the day after use.[41] Short-term use, if at all, should be advocated.

Melatonin appears to be relatively safe as an over-the-counter sleep aid; however, there are concerns about purity of preparations and variations of actual dose per pill, as these are not overseen by the U.S. Food and Drug Administration.

What We Can Do to Improve Our Sleep

We should do what we can to stabilize our circadian rhythm by following routines and avoiding circadian rhythm disturbances such as evening use of artificial light and screens. Use of light emitting ebooks and tablets before sleep has been shown to suppress melatonin, cause delayed circadian rhythm, and impact morning alertness,[42,43] but these side effects can be minimized by the addition of a blue-light filter to the screen or wearing blue light filter glasses. We should avoid or modulate intake of substances such as caffeine and alcohol for better quality sleep. We can try non-substance sleep aids such as teas without caffeine, hot baths prior to bedtime, dark and quiet rooms (or white noise instruments), and room temperature optimization (cooler is better than warmer). We should evaluate our call schedules and limit operating after being awake for prolonged periods (eg, 24 hours) as much as possible and try to limit prolonged periods of sleep deprivation if at all possible. A conversation about the importance of sleep with your colleagues and with administrators may help us shift the culture toward one where we prioritize the importance of sleep. These authors feel that this is one of the most important aspects of well-being that our culture has overlooked. Knowing our limits and identifying the effects of sleep deprivation on ourselves and colleagues must be encouraged. We need to learn to call for help when needed and respond appropriately when asked for help.

Box 1 lists suggestions to improve the quality of your sleep.

NUTRITION

Surprisingly, or not, physicians frequently do not eat well. A study published in 2004 of male physicians

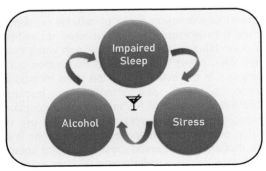

Fig. 2. Alcohol sleep disorder.

revealed that 44% of them were overweight and 6% were obese.[44] A Medscape Physician Lifestyle report 10 years later (in 2014) noted that almost 50% of surgeons were overweight, similar to the trend of increasing obesity in the US population. In this Medscape study, surgeons were the most overweight of all specialties studied. Clearly, we have somewhat neglected the importance of proper nutrition, although there are many reasons for the overweight physician population. Sleep deprivation has many negative effects on our metabolism and our eating habits. Chronic partial sleep loss increases the risk for weight gain and obesity.[45] Multiple experiments have shown that sleep restriction has profound effects such as decreased glucose tolerance, decreased insulin sensitivity, increased evening concentrations of cortisol, increased levels of ghrelin, decreased levels of leptin, and increased hunger and appetite.[46,47] It makes sense that after an all-night operation that donut in the breakroom looks and tastes so good! An understanding of these changes in our endocrine and metabolic systems may help us control the food that we do eat in these times of stress (**Fig. 3**).

Eating 3 healthy meals a day is an exception for most of CT surgeons. Many of us skip breakfast to get our day rolling, relying on the stimulation of caffeine and the energy of last night's meal. Missing breakfast has been shown in some studies to have a negative effect on endocrine and glycemic control.[48] Many forego a healthy lunch as well for various reasons and rely on a large evening meal which is suboptimal as late, large meals have been shown to increase weight gain. A randomized clinical trial revealed that late dinner induces nighttime glucose intolerance[49] and is associated with obesity,[50] hyperglycemia,[51] and dyslipidemia.[52]

While a full description of CT surgeons' eating habits is not available, we all have enough knowledge to see the low hanging fruit (pun intended) to improve our diet. Reviewing our habits and improving our intake of healthy foods such as fruit and vegetables and limiting our consumption of unhealthy foods is within the control of all of us.

It appears as if we as surgeons also neglect to keep ourselves adequately hydrated. A survey at Mayo clinic revealed that physicians who worked in operating rooms had the highest prevalence of kidney stones out of all health care workers with a rate of 17.4%.[53] Access to drinking water is usually easily available throughout our hospitals, so improved hydration is a simple improvement with great benefit.

Vitamin D deficiency is common in medical doctors due to long indoor work hours and decreased sun-exposure. One study has found that 90% of medical students were vitamin D deficient,[54] and another study showed rates of deficiency of 79% to 88% in medical doctors.[55] While these studies were performed in India, a recent study has shown that more than 50% of practicing physicians are vitamin D deficient in North America.[56] Vitamin D is essential for bone and mental health and deficient levels play a role in the development of osteoarthritis and stress fractures[57] and have been associated with depression.[58] With the high incidence of back and neck problems (70%) seen in CT surgeons in the United States,[59] CT surgeons must ensure adequate sun exposure or consider vitamin D supplementation.

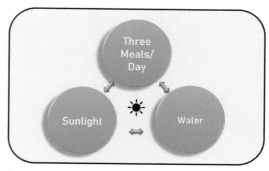

Fig. 3. Wellness.

Prolonged standing increases risk and exacerbates the development of varicose veins,[60,61] and the odds of having varicose veins increases 27-fold with every additional hour of standing per day.[62] CT surgeons routinely stand for prolonged periods of time as their typical cases are long. Recognizing this factor early in one's career and taking precautions to wear compressive stockings if necessary for long cases (or routinely) can help mitigate varicose vein pain and detrimental limitations.

HEALTH MAINTENANCE

CT surgeons must not forget to take care of those things we recommend to our own patients: regular exercise, routine medical checkups, and regular visits to the dentist (**Fig. 4**).

To endure prolonged periods and repetitive stress on the lower neck, back, knees and ankles, CT surgeons must maintain and optimize their physical health. Maintaining a healthy body mass index will tremendously maximize the longevity of the spine and joints as obesity is related to lower back pain[63] and musculoskeletal and joint pain.[64–66] Additionally, obesity is linked to osteoarthritis and related pain.[67] Diet and exercise have been shown to reduce the severity of symptoms in osteoarthritis patients.[68] Regular exercise, weight control, and favorable posture can increase the longevity of the skeletal system. Musculoskeletal pain can be detrimental to patient care: Pain can cause reduced sustained focus, reduced/restricted movements, and increased unnecessary hastiness due to physician discomfort.

In a 2022 survey of American Association for Thoracic Surgery (AATS) members, less than half of the 664 respondents reported exercising as often as they recommend for their patients.[59] Regular exercise is one of the healthiest ways to maintain a healthy body weight (when combined with adequate and healthy eating habits). More importantly for CT surgeons, activity that includes a balance of aerobic training and maintenance of strength, mobility, and flexibility allows us to meet the physical demands of our daily jobs in the operating room while optimizing the sustainability of a career that involves more "manual labor" than that of our non-surgeon counterparts in medicine. Moreover, the structure of a regular exercise routine provides the framework for groundedness that optimizes the focus, performance, and mental and physical well-being of a surgeon.[69] Including 30 minutes for some physical activity daily as a break (even just a brisk walk) can replenish precious attentional resources that allow for better decision-making and increased productivity when performing the more difficult tasks required of a CT surgeon.[70]

Combining exercise with social interactions with family and friends such as exercising with a close one or holding a casual conversation during exercise time can help overcome the monotony of exercising and can make for efficient use of time as previously mentioned. Exercising with the goal of health maintenance rather than increasing muscle mass or improving physical esthetics is central to setting an achievable goal from exercise routines. This will encourage persistence and avoid demoralization.

To optimize joint preservation, one must focus on exercises that are not taxing on joints and tendons. Choosing low impact and high repetition activities maintains healthy joints for the long run. A few examples of low-stress exercises include brisk walking, swimming, deep water running, cycling, and the use of elliptical machines rather than treadmills for running to avoid repetitive trauma to the knees and ankles. Of course, inclusion of a wide variety of activities would be ideal to break monotony and build different muscle groups. This avoids the perception of exercising as being burdensome.

Massage, physical therapy, and yoga may also help improve musculoskeletal integrity. Yoga may be useful for treatment and prevention of occupational musculoskeletal problems.[71] However, yoga was not found to relieve lower back pain according to a Cochrane database systematic review.[72] Physical therapy and massage also have roles in treating lower back pain.[73] These modalities have varying degrees of benefit, and results vary by individual, but many surgeons use such adjuncts for maintenance of musculoskeletal health and longevity.

Further tips and tricks for health maintenance are found in **Box 2**.

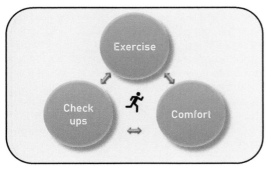

Fig. 4. Well-being.

CLOSING STATEMENT

This article is a reminder for all of us in this profession to take a step back and reassess the high

---

Box 2
Further tips and tricks for health maintenance

1. Use comfortable shoes at work and outside to avoid pain in soles of feet (from plantar fasciitis and other conditions).

2. Establish proper positioning for your surgical loops to decrease neck pain and risk of chronic neck injury.

3. Check vision before getting new loupes.

4. Perform frequent posture adjustments during long cases and optimize ergonomics (as discussed in ergonomics article).

5. Aim for at least one physical activity per day for at least 30 minutes and avoid overextending oneself to avoid excessive fatigue.

Current CDC recommendation is 150 minutes of exercise per week.

6. Focus on intermittent activities or hobbies that help replenish your cognitive resources and relieve stress for mini-breaks on a regular basis.

---

points of well-being starting with sleep, nutrition, health maintenance, and exercise. Working on this article made us reassess our habits and reminded us that maintaining our well-being is central to the care we provide for our patients. We hope that it will benefit readers similarly.

DISCLOSURE

The authors of the article have no disclosure of any commercial or financial conflict of interest pertaining to this work.

REFERENCES

1. Ruiz FS, Andersen ML, Martins RC, et al. Immune alterations after selective rapid eye movement or total sleep deprivation in healthy male volunteers. Innate Immun 2012;18(1):44–54.

2. Palagini L, Bruno RM, Gemignani A, et al. Sleep loss and hypertension: a systematic review. Curr Pharmaceut Des 2013;19(13):2409–19.

3. Tobaldini E, Fiorelli EM, Solbiati M, et al. Short sleep duration and cardiometabolic risk: from pathophysiology to clinical evidence. Nat Rev Cardiol 2019; 16(4):213–24.

4. Institute of Medicine (US) Committee on Sleep Medicine and Research. In: Colten HR, Altevogt BM, editors. Sleep Disorders and Sleep Deprivation: An Unmet Public Health Problem. National Academies Press (US); Washington, DC, 2006.

5. Walker MP, Stickgold R. Sleep-dependent learning and memory consolidation. Neuron 2004;44(1): 121–33.

6. Ackermann S, Rasch B. Differential effects of non-REM and REM sleep on memory consolidation? Curr Neurol Neurosci Rep 2014;14(2):430.

7. Walker MP, Brakefield T, Morgan A, et al. Practice with sleep makes perfect: sleep-dependent motor skill learning. Neuron 2002;35(1):205–11.

8. Wang YQ, Liu WY, Li L, et al. Neural circuitry underlying REM sleep: A review of the literature and current concepts. Prog Neurobiol 2021;204:102106.

9. Peever J, Fuller PM. The Biology of REM Sleep. Curr Biol : CB 2017;27(22):R1237–48.

10. Barbato G. REM Sleep: An Unknown Indicator of Sleep Quality. Int J Environ Res Public Health 2021; 18(24).

11. Walker MP. Why we sleep: unlocking the power of sleep and dreams. Simon and Schuster; 2017.

12. Blumberg MS, Coleman CM, Gerth AI, et al. Spatiotemporal structure of REM sleep twitching reveals developmental origins of motor synergies. Curr Biol : CB 2013;23(21):2100–9.

13. Brooks PL, Peever J. A Temporally Controlled Inhibitory Drive Coordinates Twitch Movements during REM Sleep. Curr Biol : CB 2016;26(9):1177–82.

14. Van Dongen HP, Maislin G, Mullington JM, et al. The cumulative cost of additional wakefulness: dose-response effects on neurobehavioral functions and sleep physiology from chronic sleep restriction and total sleep deprivation. Sleep 2003;26(2):117–26.

15. Williamson AM, Feyer AM. Moderate sleep deprivation produces impairments in cognitive and motor performance equivalent to legally prescribed levels of alcohol intoxication. Occup Environ Med 2000; 57(10):649–55.

16. Mohtashami F, Thiele A, Karreman E, et al. Comparing technical dexterity of sleep-deprived versus intoxicated surgeons. J Soc Laparoendosc Surg 2014;18(4).

17. Banfi T, Coletto E, d'Ascanio P, et al. Effects of Sleep Deprivation on Surgeons Dexterity. Front Neurol 2019;10:595.

18. Taffinder NJ, McManus IC, Gul Y, et al. Effect of sleep deprivation on surgeons' dexterity on laparoscopy simulator. Lancet 1998;352(9135):1191.

19. Growdon W, Ghika J, Henderson J, et al. Effects of proximal and distal muscles' groups contraction and mental stress on the amplitude and frequency of physiological finger tremor. An accelerometric study. Electromyogr Clin Neurophysiol 2000;40(5): 295–303.

20. Basaran K, Mercan ES, Aygit AC. Effects of Fatigue and Sleep Deprivation on Microvascular Anastomoses. J Craniofac Surg 2015;26(4):1342–7.

21. Uchal M, Tjugum J, Martinsen E, et al. The impact of sleep deprivation on product quality and procedure

effectiveness in a laparoscopic physical simulator: a randomized controlled trial. Am J Surg 2005;189(6):753–7.

22. Tomasko JM, Pauli EM, Kunselman AR, et al. Sleep deprivation increases cognitive workload during simulated surgical tasks. Am J Surg 2012;203(1):37–43.

23. Jakubowicz DM, Price EM, Glassman HJ, et al. Effects of a twenty-four hour call period on resident performance during simulated endoscopic sinus surgery in an accreditation council for graduate medical education-compliant training program. Laryngoscope 2005;115(1):143–6.

24. Leff DR, Aggarwal R, Rana M, et al. Laparoscopic skills suffer on the first shift of sequential night shifts: program directors beware and residents prepare. Ann Surg 2008;247(3):530–9.

25. Whelehan DF, Alexander M, Connelly TM, et al. Sleepy Surgeons: A Multi-Method Assessment of Sleep Deprivation and Performance in Surgery. J Surg Res 2021;268:145–57.

26. Coleman JJ, Robinson CK, Zarzaur BL, et al. To Sleep, Perchance to Dream: Acute and Chronic Sleep Deprivation in Acute Care Surgeons. J Am Coll Surg 2019;229(2):166–74.

27. Yang Z, Takahashi T, Gerull WD, et al. Impact of Nighttime Lung Transplantation on Outcomes and Costs. Ann Thorac Surg 2021;112(1):206–13.

28. Mitchell DC, Knight CA, Hockenberry J, et al. Beverage caffeine intakes in the U.S. Food Chem Toxicol 2014;63:136–42.

29. Clark I, Landolt HP. Coffee, caffeine, and sleep: A systematic review of epidemiological studies and randomized controlled trials. Sleep Med Rev 2017;31:70–8.

30. Karacan I, Thornby JI, Anch M, et al. Dose-related sleep disturbances induced by coffee and caffeine. Clin Pharmacol Ther 1976;20(6):682–9.

31. Aggarwal R, Mishra A, Crochet P, et al. Effect of caffeine and taurine on simulated laparoscopy performed following sleep deprivation. Br J Surg 2011;98(11):1666–72.

32. Urso-Baiarda F, Shurey S, Grobbelaar AO. Effect of caffeine on microsurgical technical performance. Microsurgery 2007;27(2):84–7.

33. O'Callaghan F, Muurlink O, Reid N. Effects of caffeine on sleep quality and daytime functioning. Risk Manag Healthc Pol 2018;11:263–71.

34. Thakkar MM, Sharma R, Sahota P. Alcohol disrupts sleep homeostasis. Alcohol 2015;49(4):299–310.

35. Payerchin R. Survey: 1 in 7 physicians use alcohol, drugs while on the job to cope with stress. 2022. Available at: https://www.medicaleconomics.com/view/survey-1-in-7-physicians-use-alcohol-drugs-while-on-the-job-to-cope-with-stress.

36. Oreskovich MR, Kaups KL, Balch CM, et al. Prevalence of alcohol use disorders among American surgeons. Arch Surg 2012;147(2):168–74.

37. Brower KJ, Perron BE. Sleep disturbance as a universal risk factor for relapse in addictions to psychoactive substances. Med Hypotheses 2010;74(5):928–33.

38. de Mendonca FMR, de Mendonca G, Souza LC, et al. Benzodiazepines and Sleep Architecture: A Systematic Review. CNS Neurol Disord - Drug Targets 2023;22(2):172–9.

39. Guilleminault C. Benzodiazepines, breathing, and sleep. Am J Med 1990;88(3A):25S–8S.

40. Lane SD, Tcheremissine OV, Lieving LM, et al. Acute effects of alprazolam on risky decision making in humans. Psychopharmacology (Berl) 2005;181(2):364–73.

41. Ozdemir PG, Karadag AS, Selvi Y, et al. Assessment of the effects of antihistamine drugs on mood, sleep quality, sleepiness, and dream anxiety. Int J Psychiatr Clin Pract 2014;18(3):161–8.

42. Chang AM, Aeschbach D, Duffy JF, et al. Evening use of light-emitting eReaders negatively affects sleep, circadian timing, and next-morning alertness. Proc Natl Acad Sci USA 2015;112(4):1232–7.

43. Chinoy ED, Duffy JF, Czeisler CA. Unrestricted evening use of light-emitting tablet computers delays self-selected bedtime and disrupts circadian timing and alertness. Phys Rep 2018;6(10):e13692.

44. Ajani UA, Lotufo PA, Gaziano JM, et al. Body mass index and mortality among US male physicians. Ann Epidemiol 2004;14(10):731–9.

45. Reutrakul S, Van Cauter E. Sleep influences on obesity, insulin resistance, and risk of type 2 diabetes. Metabolism 2018;84:56–66.

46. Koren D, Taveras EM. Association of sleep disturbances with obesity, insulin resistance and the metabolic syndrome. Metabolism 2018;84:67–75.

47. Antza C, Kostopoulos G, Mostafa S, et al. The links between sleep duration, obesity and type 2 diabetes mellitus. J Endocrinol 2021;252(2):125–41.

48. Chowdhury EA, Richardson JD, Tsintzas K, et al. Carbohydrate-rich breakfast attenuates glycaemic, insulinaemic and ghrelin response to ad libitum lunch relative to morning fasting in lean adults. Br J Nutr 2015;114(1):98–107.

49. Tomura S, Chida Y, Ida T, et al. Platelet adenine nucleotides in patients with primary glomerular disease. Tohoku J Exp Med 1988;156(3):221–7.

50. Xiao Q, Garaulet M, Scheer F. Meal timing and obesity: interactions with macronutrient intake and chronotype. Int J Obes 2019;43(9):1701–11.

51. Nakajima K, Suwa K. Association of hyperglycemia in a general Japanese population with late-night-dinner eating alone, but not breakfast skipping alone. J Diabetes Metab Disord 2015;14:16.

52. Yoshida J, Eguchi E, Nagaoka K, et al. Association of night eating habits with metabolic syndrome and its components: a longitudinal study. BMC Publ Health 2018;18(1):1366.

53. Linder B. Title: Kidney stones prove occupational hazard for surgeons, mayo clinic study finds. 2013.

Available at: https://newsnetwork.mayoclinic.org/discussion/kidney-stones-prove-occupational-hazard-for-surgeons-mayo-clinic-study-finds/.

54. Nadeem S, Munim TF, Hussain HF, et al. Determinants of Vitamin D deficiency in asymptomatic healthy young medical students. Pakistan J Med Sci 2018;34(5):1248–52.

55. Sudheesh S, Boaz RJ. Degrees of Deficiency: Doctors and Vitamin D. Indian J Community Med 2017; 42(1):53.

56. Sowah D, Fan X, Dennett L, et al. Vitamin D levels and deficiency with different occupations: a systematic review. BMC Publ Health 2017;17(1):519.

57. Christodoulou S, Goula T, Ververidis A, et al. Vitamin D and bone disease. BioMed Res Int 2013;2013: 396541.

58. Anglin RE, Samaan Z, Walter SD, et al. Vitamin D deficiency and depression in adults: systematic review and meta-analysis. Br J Psychiatry 2013;202: 100–7.

59. Bremner RM, Ungerleider RM, Ungerleider J, et al. Well-being of Cardiothoracic Surgeons in the Time of COVID-19: A Survey by the Wellness Committee of the American Association for Thoracic Surgery. Semin Thorac Cardiovasc Surg 2024;36(1):129–36.

60. Tuchsen F, Hannerz H, Burr H, et al. Prolonged standing at work and hospitalisation due to varicose veins: a 12 year prospective study of the Danish population. Occup Environ Med 2005;62(12):847–50.

61. Tuchsen F, Krause N, Hannerz H, et al. Standing at work and varicose veins. Scand J Work Environ Health 2000;26(5):414–20.

62. Shakya R, Karmacharya RM, Shrestha R, et al. Varicose veins and its risk factors among nurses at Dhulikhel hospital: a cross sectional study. BMC Nurs 2020;19:8.

63. Lucha-Lopez MO, Hidalgo-Garcia C, Monti-Ballano S, et al. Body Mass Index and Its Influence on Chronic Low Back Pain in the Spanish Population: A Secondary Analysis from the European Health Survey (2020). Biomedicines 2023;11(8).

64. Krul M, van der Wouden JC, Schellevis FG, et al. Musculoskeletal problems in overweight and obese children. Ann Fam Med 2009;7(4):352–6.

65. Deere KC, Clinch J, Holliday K, et al. Obesity is a risk factor for musculoskeletal pain in adolescents: findings from a population-based cohort. Pain 2012;153(9):1932–8.

66. Vennu V, Alenazi AM, Abdulrahman TA, et al. Obesity and Multisite Pain in the Lower Limbs: Data from the Osteoarthritis Initiative. Pain Res Manag 2020;2020:6263505.

67. Bliddal H, Leeds AR, Christensen R. Osteoarthritis, obesity and weight loss: evidence, hypotheses and horizons - a scoping review. Obes Rev 2014;15(7): 578–86.

68. Messier SP, Loeser RF, Miller GD, et al. Exercise and dietary weight loss in overweight and obese older adults with knee osteoarthritis: the Arthritis, Diet, and Activity Promotion Trial. Arthritis Rheum 2004; 50(5):1501–10.

69. Stulberg B. The practice of groundedness: a transformative path to success that feeds–not crushes– your soul. Penguin Publishing Group; 2021.

70. Attention span: a groundbreaking way to restore balance, happiness and productivity. Hanover Square Press; 2023.

71. Gandolfi MG, Zamparini F, Spinelli A, et al. Asana for Neck, Shoulders, and Wrists to Prevent Musculoskeletal Disorders among Dental Professionals: In-Office Yoga Protocol. J Funct Morphol Kinesiol 2023;8(1).

72. Wieland LS, Skoetz N, Pilkington K, et al. Yoga for chronic non-specific low back pain. Cochrane Database Syst Rev 2022;11(11):CD010671.

73. Kim TH, Park SK, Cho IY, et al. Substantiating the Therapeutic Effects of Simultaneous Heat Massage Combined with Conventional Physical Therapy for Treatment of Lower Back Pain: A Randomized Controlled Feasibility Trial. Healthcare (Basel) 2023; 11(7).

Financial Well-Being for Thoracic Surgeons

Louis F. Chai, MD[a], Michael P. Salna, MD, MBA[b], Bryan Payne Stanifer, MD, MPH[c],*

KEYWORDS

- Wellness • Financial literacy • Student loans • Insurance • Investment • Asset management
- Cardiothoracic surgery

KEY POINTS

- There are 5 types of student loans, each with unique qualifications, interest rates, repayment plans, and opportunities for loan forgiveness.
- Educational funds can be obtained from multiple sources and can be accrued from the moment a child is born.
- Building financial strength can be accomplished using a diversified portfolio and can be highly individualized based on stage of career, short- and long-term goals, and opportunities available.
- Protection of accumulated assets is critical and can be accomplished with insurance, wills, and estate planning to provide current and future coverage.

INTRODUCTION

Financial well-being is an essential part of overall wellness, affording the freedom to enjoy life, and focus on other priorities. This is a complex topic and what follows is a brief, but comprehensive overview of education financing, investing, as well as retirement and estate planning.

Financing Undergraduate and Medical School Education

Educational savings can start from the moment a child is born. With average tuition increasing more than $15,000 annually, few can afford the costs without financial aid (FA), commonly through student loans and educational funds.[1]

STUDENT LOANS
Federal

Comprising 92% of student debt, federal loans are distributed through the Department of Education with loan servicers collecting repayments. Eligibility is determined by the Free Application for Federal Student Aid (FAFSA) and 4 options are available: direct subsidized loan (DSL), direct unsubsidized loan (DUL), direct parent loan for undergraduate students (PLUS), and direct consolidation loan (DCL). General benefits are lower and subsidized interest rates, deferment periods, diverse repayment options, and forgiving delinquency policies (**Table 1**).[2–6]

Direct subsidized loan

Federal direct loans are considered the most favorable and can be subsidized or unsubsidized.

The DSL is for undergraduates with "need-based aid" determined as the difference between cost of attendance (COA) and expected family contribution.[7] There are limits to DSLs that students are eligible for annually and in total as determined by the FAFSA, COA, other FA, year in school, and dependency status. This is also a combined limit between DSLs and DULs.

[a] Department of Thoracic Medicine and Surgery, Temple University Hospital, 3401 North Broad Street, Suite 501-C, Philadelphia, PA 19140, USA; [b] Department of Surgery, Division of Cardiac, Thoracic, and Vascular Surgery, Columbia University Medical Center, 177 Fort Washington, 7-435, New York, NY 10032, USA; [c] Department of Surgery, Division of Cardiac, Thoracic, and Vascular Surgery, Columbia University Medical Center, 161 Fort Washington Avenue, 3rd Floor, New York, NY 10032, USA
* Corresponding author.
E-mail address: bps2131@cumc.columbia.edu

Thorac Surg Clin 34 (2024) 223–232
https://doi.org/10.1016/j.thorsurg.2024.04.010
1547-4127/24/© 2024 Elsevier Inc. All rights are reserved, including those for text and data mining, AI training, and similar technologies.

Table 1
Option of Federal loans distribution

	Direct Subsidized	Direct Unsubsidized	Direct PLUSlus	Direct Consolidation	Private
Credit heck	Not required	Not required	Required[a]	Not required	Required
Interest Rates	Fixed	Fixed [b]	Fixed	Weighted	Fixed
Loan Forgiveness	Yes	Yes	GPLs – Yes PPL – Consolidation required	Yes	No
Deferment Periods	Yes	Yes[c]	GPL – Yes PPL – Approval required	Yes	No

[a] Can still obtain with co-signer or endorser with good credit.
[b] Different rates for graduates and undergraduates.
[c] Interest accrues during deferment periods.

One DSL advantage is it is annually adjusted with fixed interest rates. They have been fairly stable over the past decade between 3% and 5%.[8] One key difference between the DSLs and other loans is the Investors Relation is covered by the government during defined periods –enrollment at least half time, the 6-month grace period after graduating, and during deferment periods. This is a huge benefit as interest does not accrue while in school and reduces debt by removing additional interest to be repaid or compounded principal.

However, DSLs have associated fees. The major fee is the origination fee, which is charged as a fixed percentage of the total loan amount by the lender for issuing the loan. This is deducted from loan disbursements, reducing the amount received compared with the amount approved to borrow. Consequently, repayment amounts increases because it includes the borrowed amount with origination fees and accrued interest resulting in students repaying more than received.[9] Fortunately, origination fees for DSLs are low compared with other federal loans.[10]

In terms of repayment, deferment can occur during the aforementioned defined periods. After the grace period, repayment begins and is handled by loan servicers.[11] DSLs are eligible for income-driven repayment (IDR) plans with potential loan forgiveness through programs like Public Service Loan Forgiveness (PSLF).

Direct unsubsidized loans
DULs are available to undergraduates and graduates and are similar to DSLs, but some crucial differences make them less favorable.

DUL qualification is categorized as "non-need-based aid." This only considers COA and how much aid has already been obtained with non-need-based aid being the difference between the 2. DUL is one option to fulfill that difference.[6,7]

The second difference pertains to the interest. Unlike DSL, loan interest accrues when the loan is received, regardless of active payment phase or not. This is critical for graduate students because their DUL has higher interest rates compared with undergraduates and because they defer payment for continued schooling, the total repayment amount increases to significantly more than the original loan. Thus, while graduate students can obtain DULs, this interest accruement may make DULs less attractive.

Direct parent loan for undergraduate students
Direct PLUS loans (DPLs)s are broken into Grad PLUS Loans (GPLs) and Parent PLUS Loans (PPLs). GPLs are available for graduate students while PPLs are for parents of dependent undergraduates. Both fill gaps after DSLs and DULs are maximized and out of pocket payments are made.[6]

DPL terms are less favorable than other federal loans. Rates are fixed, but significantly higher annually compared with DSLs and DULs. DPLs also come with origination fees, further increasing repayment amounts.

GPLs and PPLs differ in repayment terms. Both may disburse up to the COA, but repayments are expected at different times. GPL borrowers have deferment periods as mentioned earlier while PPL borrowers begin repayments as soon as the loan is disbursed or must apply for deferment. In terms of repayment plans, GPLs qualify for IDR or PSLF, but PPLs must apply for consolidation to qualify or extend payments over longer periods to lower monthly payments.

Direct consolidation loans
DCLs are not unique loans, but an option to combine qualifying federal loans after schooling is complete.

Consolidation offers several advantages. Logistically, consolidation simplifies things into 1 loan and servicer rather than multiple with different repayment schedules and accounts, fees, and potential missed payments. Fiscally, interest is combined in a weighted fashion (rounded up to the nearest 1/8%). This may reduce payments long-term on high-interest loans, but low-interest loans may cost more so careful consideration must be taken when deciding which loans to combine and whether it makes fiscal sense over the repayment term.

DCLs are eligible for IDRs and PSLF. When terms are met, the remaining debt is released, reducing final payoff amounts. However, if any consolidated loans previously met PSLF or IDR terms, the credit is lost as DCLs are considered a "different" loan. Again, careful consideration is required to maximize fiscal savings and weighing different payment options.

Private

Private loans (PLs) comprise 8% of borrower debt. They come from multiple sources and can be standalone or supplement federal loans.[3,12,13] While they function similarly to federal loans, there are distinct advantages and disadvantages.

One advantage is higher loan limits. While federal loans can be capped, PLs typically allow up to COA. This may simplify the borrowing and repayment logistics, rather than multiple federal loans to meet total need.

Another advantage is in repayments. PL rates can be significantly lower than federal loans. Those with low-interest PLs that make payments quickly may save money long-term by avoiding buildup of unpaid interest. The repayment timeframes are more variable (5–20 years) and are loaner dependent compared with the standard federal loan 10 years.[14] However, there are no IDR or forgiveness programs to minimize monthly payments as with federal loans. PLs have defined payment schedules to follow to avoid defaulting and those that qualify for PLs must be sure they can afford repayment before applying.

Disadvantages to PLs include a credit approval requirement, limiting access as many students have not built-up credit. However, PLs may still be obtained with a co-signer. Finally, those with worse credit scores that are approved have higher interest rates, negating 1 major benefit of PLs.

Additionally, the multitude of PLs require more work and personal time to find suitable loans whereas Federal loans provide a streamlined process where eligibility and loan amounts are determined by the FAFSA.

EDUCATION FUNDS
529 Plans

529 plans (529s), or "qualified tuition plans", are a fund option for college education investments, K-12 education, payoffs for student loans, and to fund Roth Individual Retirement Accounts (IRAs).[15,16]

529s are offered by individual states, though there is no residency requirement to apply. Some offer unique benefits for in-state residents that are often a tax-break but some offer monetary bonuses or contributions when opening an account. Withdrawals are tax-free when used for the designed purposes and accounts are not included in the owner's assets.[17] 529s are broken into education savings plans (ESP) and prepaid tuition plans (PTP).

ESPs are investment accounts to accumulate money for future educational expenses including tuition, room and board, or loan repayments.[18] ESPs function like standard investment accounts with a customizable investment portfolio that can be tailored based on when money is needed; those needing it sooner (eg, elementary or secondary school) may choose low-risk options to prevent investment loss whereas long-term needs have time to recover from losses in riskier investments.

Alternatively, PTPs provide credits for the future. The principal benefit is to combat the rising COA each year.[19] Investors purchase credits at the current prices that can then be used for future classes at no additional cost. PTP credits must be used at participating institutions in the state that sponsored the plan and for tuition and mandatory fees, limiting flexibility compared with ESPs. Credits may still be used to pay for alternative institutions, albeit worth smaller amounts than initial purchase value. Additional risk comes from sponsor financial failure, resulting in partial or complete loss of credits.[18]

One disadvantage is the associated costs. Both ESPs and PTPs may have application fees and annual account administrative fees. ESPs also have additional charges such as general and asset management and trading fees. On reviewing these, it is critical to determine which plan is right for individuals to avoid unnecessary losses. Additionally, 529s may also impact eligibility for need-based FA. Finally, some degree of investor financial literacy is paramount to maximize growth, limit excess fees, and appropriately use funds.

Scholarships

Scholarships vary in award amount and qualifications with the majority being merit-based and do not require repayment. They are offered by government, for-profit companies, non-profit organizations, and educational institutions at all levels of education. Some criteria for earning scholarships include grade point averages and standardized test scores, community service, athletic success, gender, cultural or ethnic background, participation in the military, or disability.[20] There is no limit on number of applications, but it can be labor intensive and highly competitive. In addition, earning scholarships impacts FA so understanding the application deadlines and notifications of approval are important to avoid excess borrowing.[21]

Grants

Similarly, grants are based on specific eligibility criteria and can come from many sources.[20] Government grants can be a part of the FAFSA-determined FA package. Grants usually do not require repayment unless certain stipulations are not met; in these scenarios, penalties include conversion to an interest-bearing loan or ineligibility for further FA.[22] Thus, grants represent a source of debt-free funds for education but require an organized process to maximize and maintain opportunities.

Work Study

Work study is a government program through which eligibility is determined by the FAFSA and based on financial need. Eligible individuals work in part-time jobs at their educational institution to earn stipends awarded in the FA package.[23] Payment is through a paycheck dispersed at designated intervals, rather than lump sum distribution like other FA, but requires students to find eligible positions and work the required hours to earn the money. The jobs vary, but generally focus on community service and when possible, relate to the field of study. The program is limited in overall amount and availability but helps defray costs and allows some flexibility with spending money for non-educational obligations such as housing.

BUILDING FINANCIAL STRENGTH, INCREASING PERSONAL ASSETS, AND PLANNING FOR RETIREMENT
Investments

While structuring investments is important, optimizing your investment tax strategy is even more important. This will allow you to take fewer risks on your investments and still net more money.

Taxes will be discussed in more details in the Retirement section but for now, there are 2 categories of investment taxes: income and capital gains. Income tax carries the highest tax rate. Capital gains tax refers to taxation on gains you made through appreciation of investments. If an investment is held for less than 1 year, any gains made are considered *short-term* and taxed as ordinary income. However, if an investment is held longer than 1 year, the rate is much lower (regardless of your income bracket; the top capital gains tax bracket is only 20% for incomes higher than $492,300). It stands to reason, then, that you want to optimize your long-term capital gains taxes and reduce income taxes.

Stocks

The short-run performance of the stock market is unpredictable. There is a high probability that your stock picks will not beat the aggregate returns of the market. This is one reason why portfolio managers are not paid solely based on their returns. The 2022 S&P Indices versus Active scorecard, which tracks actively managed fund performance against their respective category benchmarks showed that nearly 80% of fund managers underperformed the S&P.[24]

This means that you probably would have been better off investing $1 in every company in the S&P 500 than $500 on the newest biotech startup. Index funds are an investment vehicle that attempt to recreate the make-up and thereby match the returns of a segment of the market. For example, Vanguard's 500 Index tracks the performance of the S&P 500 by holding shares in all of these companies. This diversification reduces the volatility risk in any given sector (eg, energy, finance, or technology) and greatly simplifies investment decisions. In general, you should have a very compelling reason for investing in individual stocks over an index fund or exchange-traded fund (ETF).

ETFs are very similar to index funds in that they are a basket of stocks in a given sector or index *except* they can be bought and sold throughout the day like stocks.

Bonds

Bonds are pieces of debt, issued by governments or companies that are sold to investors. Like any type of loan, there is a fixed lifespan of the loan at which point the bond must be paid back, as well as interest payments to the bond holder for loaning this money.

Mutual Funds

Mutual funds are traditionally run by a portfolio manager who actively buys and sells shares using 'mutually' pooled money from investors. In general, these active funds tend to underperform passive index funds and have quite a few costs associated with them (refer to aforementioned section). There are passive, index mutual funds, however.

Cash

It may feel good to see a lot of cash in your checking account, but you are automatically giving up 2% to 3% of annual purchasing power to inflation. There is no upside to holding lots of cash, only guaranteed downside.

Asset allocation

Most of your portfolio's returns will come from your asset allocation – the percentage breakdown in different asset classes (from stocks to bonds to real estate). Since the authors discussed earlier that you are best off simply investing in passive index funds – most of your time should be focused on these allocation ratios rather than hunting for the next stock winner.

In general, you should be diversified in domestic stocks, international stocks, bonds, and other assets such as commodities or real estate. The ratios that you allocate to each of these depend on your goals, your near-term needs, and your risk tolerance. Asset allocation can get quite complicated, so it is worth discussing with a financial advisor.

RETIREMENT ACCOUNTS

Many surgeons wish they could retire but are unable to because of lifestyle creep and poor planning early in their careers. Before discussing retirement accounts, it is important to understand the difference between marginal and effective tax rates.

Marginal tax rates are often thought of as your "tax bracket" but this is just the tax rate on the next dollar you earn. Only the money in each bracket is taxed at that marginal rate. **Table 2** outlines the 2023 Federal income tax brackets for a single filer.

Effective tax is simply the amount of taxes you paid last year divided by last year's gross income. This percentage is always lower than your marginal tax rate and is more representative of your actual tax burden. Much of your income will be taxed at 10%, 12%, 22%, 24%, 32% and so on, meaning that someone with a marginal tax rate of 35% will have a much lower effective tax rate than 35%.

Growing *tax-free* means that you do not have to pay taxes each year on dividend distributions or capital gains.

Tax-deferred Accounts

Tax-deferred accounts, such as a 401(k) or traditional IRA allow you to deduct your contributions

Table 2
Outlines of the 2023 Federal income tax brackets for a single filer

Tax Rate	Taxable Income	What You Owe
10%	$0- $11,000	10% of income
12%	$11,001- $44,725	$1100 plus 12% of amount over $11,000
22%	$44,726- $95,375	$5147 plus 22% of amount over $44,725
24%	$95,376 - $182,100	$16,290 plus 24% of amount over $95,375
32%	$182,101- $231,250	$37,104 plus 32% of amount over $182,100
35%	$231,251- $578, 125	$52,832 plus 35% of amount over $231,250
37%	$578,126+	$174,238.25 plus 37% of amount over $578,125

Source: Internal Revenue Service Federal Tax Brackets. Federal income tax rates and brackets. 2023. Available at: https://www.irs.gov/filing/federal-income-tax-rates-and-brackets.

from your income up-front, have your money-grow tax-free, and then tax you at a lower rate when you pull the money out after age 59 ½. One of the great advantages of using these accounts is that you get to save at your marginal rate and pay them later at a lower effective rate.

The 2 most common employment-based tax-deferred accounts are the 401(k) and 403(b). The main difference is the type of employer sponsoring them – 401(k) plans by private, for-profit companies and 403(b) plans by nonprofit organizations and the government. Both plans have annual contribution limits (401(k) 2023 limits: $22500 or $30000 if you are older than 50).[25]

Traditional IRAs are tax-deferred retirement savings account established by an individual. While thoracic surgeons typically earn too much to be eligible to make tax-deductible contributions, anyone is allowed to contribute up to $6500 per year (in 2023) to a traditional IRA, or $7500 if you are over 50. These contributions may not be deductible, but they can still grow tax-free.[26]

A tax-free (Roth) account differs in that you contribute after-tax dollars up-front, the money grows tax-protected in the account, and is completely tax free upon withdrawal after you turn 59 ½.

After your gross income exceeds a certain limit, you can no longer contribute to a Roth IRA. In 2023, this phase-out occurs between $138000 and $153000 for single filers and $218000 and $228000 for joint filers.[27] Surgeons can still contribute through a "backdoor Roth IRA" which converts non-deductible traditional IRA contributions into a Roth IRA so that the money can grow tax-free. While not complicated, this is best done with a financial advisor.

In general, contributing to tax-deferred accounts makes the most sense during your peak earning years to capitalize on the tax arbitrage between your marginal rate at contribution and effective rate at withdrawal. In your lower earning years (residency and fellowship), these advantages are not as apparent and lower earners should focus on maximizing tax-free (Roth) contributions. This decision is more complicated for high income, high savers who may still be taxed at the highest rate in retirement. Another factor to consider is the tax regime of the state in which you work compared with the state you in which you plan to retire.

Stealth Individual Retirement Accounts or Health Savings Account

A Health Savings Account (HSA) can serve as "stealth" IRA with even greater tax benefits (though you must have a high-deductible plan to qualify). Contributions have an upfront tax deduction similar to tax-deferred retirement accounts like a 401(k), growth in the account is protected from taxation (and can be invested in stocks, bonds, or mutual funds), and withdrawals are tax-free if you spend the money on health care.[28]

ASSET LOCATION STRATEGY

Remember, when you buy a stock, real estate, or business investment outside of a retirement plan, there is no tax on that investment unless a dividend is paid or you sell. Once you sell, you will pay capital gains tax unless you sell within a year – in which case it is ordinary income taxation.

Therefore, investments which would qualify for capital gain taxation should be placed in non-retirement plan accounts. This will ensure that, assuming no significant changes to the tax code, your maximum taxation on selling these investments is only 20% long term capital gains tax.

Investments that incur ordinary income tax and have low anticipated appreciation, such as real estate investment trusts or bonds, should be put into tax-deferred or tax-free retirement accounts to shelter the annual taxation on these dividends or interest.

Mortgages

It does not always make sense to buy a home instead of renting one. Agents who justify purchasing because "the mortgage is less than your rent" are conveniently omitting the considerable expenses of home ownership and overexaggerating the tax benefits. Before committing to home ownership, you should be confident about stability your current employment. Purchase and sale of a house within a short period of time can be financially risky. Additionally, you should predict your family's future needs. Proximity to work and satellite work locations, options for quality education, and community resources are only a few considerations that influence the value of investing in a home.

Once you have made the informed decision to purchase a home, there are important considerations when evaluating mortgage options. In general, most banks will require you to put 20% of the property value down before loaning you the remaining amount as a mortgage. This is known as a down payment. Mortgages can have variable *durations*, though are typically 15- or 30-year and the longer the duration, the smaller the monthly payment (at the expense of paying more interest over the lifetime of the loan). *Rates* can either have a fixed interest rate for the entire term of the loan, or one that is *variable,* and changes based off changes in federal rates.

"DOCTOR MORTGAGES"

Banks know that physicians have high earning potential and will, therefore, offer us mortgages for which we ordinarily would not qualify. While the terms can vary by bank, in general a 'doctor mortgage' refers to a loan that requires a smaller down down payment (0%–10%) at the expense of higher interest rates and the waiver of mortgage insurance (saving you 0.6%–2% of the loan's value). These loans tend to be catered to young doctors who lack the capital to place a down payment but want to purchase a home.

PROTECTING PERSONAL ASSETS IN SCHOOL, TRAINING, LIFE, AND BEYOND
Insurance

Insurance provides a safety net of monetary coverage or reimbursement during qualifying events. In health care, there are several insurances to be familiar with: disability, life, and umbrella.

Disability

Disability insurance (DI) provides protection against unexpected events that prevents individuals from working by providing a portion of the expected income from the specific occupation. DI can be obtained from the government via the Social Security Administration (SSA), employment packages from employers, or private insurers.[29] There are a few critical concepts to understand about DI.

The first is the elimination period. This is the time between the injury or illness and when the payment benefits begin.[30] This is important as selecting an excessive elimination period may result in periods without income while selecting short elimination periods can raise upfront premiums.

Second are the benefit period and amounts. The benefit amount is the amount disbursed after the elimination period. This is calculated before taxes and is 60% of the expected income on average. However, the distribution is usually not taxed so the final income is nearly equivalent. The benefit period is the duration that the benefits last. This can range from weeks up to retirement age when social security benefits take over.[31]

Finally, "riders" are customized enhancements to DI that mainly impact policy terms and coverage rather than disbursement amounts. Important riders for physicians are "guaranteed renewable" (insurer cannot cancel a policy if premiums paid), "future purchase option" (increasing coverage after policy enactment without further screening), and "own-occupation" (receive benefits if unable to perform specific occupation, not any or all occupations).[32] Consideration of which, "riders" to add is important for different specialties and managing premiums.

The process for obtaining DI varies. Employer sponsored disability insurance (ESDI) plans are obtained during benefits enrollment. These are often part of group disability policies, more affordable, and premiums may be partially or completely covered by employers. Downsides of ESDI are limited coverage scopes and policies only apply while employed at that specific job. Social security disability insurance (SSDI) is obtained through the government via an application to the SSA. Few people are approved for SSDI given the stringent criteria and those that qualify often fall short of their necessary financial protection. Finally, private disability insurance is obtained through private companies and comes in 2 forms: short-term disability insurance (STDI) and long-term disability insurance (LTDI).

STDI is used for short coverage periods at the current job, where injury or illness prevents working, but a return-to-work is ultimately expected (eg, post-operative rehabilitation and pregnancy). STDI elimination periods are shorter (<1 month) and payouts are close to 80% of salaries.

Comparatively, LTDI is used for long-term coverage, which can be several years up to retirement. LTDI elimination periods are longer at 90 days on average and payouts are lower around 60% on most policies.[31]

After applying, the underwriting process begins that involves a physical examination and in-depth medical history to verify pre-existing medical conditions that can impact the final policy via "exclusions". These are specifications detailing prior conditions that are not covered as disabilities under the policy, regardless of the etiology of the current claims (eg, surgeon with prior neck injury has a "neck exclusion", cannot file disability claim if develops debilitating neck pain from operating). Thus, timing of obtaining DI is important as there are less likely to have exclusions when younger. In addition, some health screenings may be waived when purchasing while in training, further avoiding exclusions.[31]

Life

Life insurance (LI) is a contract between the LI company and policy holder that the insurer will pay a specified sum of money, or "death benefit", to beneficiaries when the insured passes away. Premiums can be paid at intervals or as a single upfront payment. There are 2 types of LI that differ based on coverage duration.[33]

Term life insurance (TLI) covers predetermined timeframes chosen at policy enactment. TLI weighs the affordability of premiums to guarantee a death benefit to long-term financial strength. For example, in the event of an early death where the insured did not have significant assets built up, the additional death benefit may provide extra security, but an older person may have accumulated enough resources without the need for an additional payout.

TLI is further broken into subtypes. Renewable TLI is a policy that is renewed annually with a new and higher quote to account for the increased risk with older age. Alternatively, convertible TLI allows policyholders to convert TLIs into permanent life insurance (PLI).

PLI provides similar benefits but covers the entire life and is correspondingly more expensive. The most common PLI subtype is whole LI. This policy has stable premium of which a portion contributes to a cash value component that grows over time at fixed rates.[34] Once enough value is accumulated, money can be withdrawn to pay premiums or used with no payback requirement. However, any amount withdrawn beyond the expected death benefit is deducted from the beneficiaries' disbursement. Other subtypes are universal, indexed universal, and variable universal LI which are all similar, but differ in premiums, cash value component functionality, and death benefit amounts.

Umbrella

Umbrella insurance (UI) provides additional liability coverage beyond existing policies for an additional premium. This affords additional asset protection to cover on top of what individual policies offer. UI extends globally, but requires policyholders to carry other specific policies, particularly auto and property given the high risk for personal liability.[35]

ESTATE PLANNING

Nobody lives forever. Estate planning is essential to control what happens to your assets when you die and having a strategy in place could mean less estate and income taxes for your loved ones when that time comes.

First, you will need a will that dictates who will manage your assets, and where they will go when you die.

Next, you want to avoid *probate* - the process whereby your will is adjudicated by a judge and your loved ones must establish their rights to your assets, even if you wrote it in your will. This is expensive, time-consuming – often requiring up to a year, and public – personal assets become public information after this process. Probate can be avoided by clearly designating beneficiaries for all accounts and assets orr using a revocable trust. There are many different types of trusts and establishing them can be complicated, so we recommend doing this with a lawyer.

A trust that is revocable means that you can remove your assets from the trust at any time. Over your lifetime you must move your assets into this trust. Revocable trusts offer very little asset protection (assets contained within them are still fair game to creditors), however, they allow heirs to receive their inheritances immediately and are generally cheaper than having a will go through probate.[36]

You should also be sure to include a "pour-over will." This ensures whatever assets you did not move into your trust before death will be 'poured' into your trust the moment you die.[37] For example, if you forget to make your trust the owner of your car, the pour-over will should remedy this oversight.

Estate and Inheritance Tax

The final piece in your strategy should be the minimization of estate and inheritance taxes. The good news is that the 2024 federal tax exemption is $13.61 (for married couples, both spouses get $13.61 M), meaning that if you die with a net worth less than this you will not pay any federal estate tax.[38]

Unfortunately, many states (mostly in the Northeast) levy their own state estate or inheritance tax burden with much lower exemption amounts (New York, for example, has a 6.58 M exemption as of 2023).[39]

The most common technique to reduce this tax burden is to give your assets away before death. There is no limit on the amount you can give to charity. When it comes to gifting to your descendants, you can make unlimited payments to medical providers or educational institutions on behalf of others (eg, granddaughter's tuition) without paying gift tax. For monetary gifts, however, you and your spouse are also allowed to gift up to $17000 per year each to as many people as you want without using up any of the estate tax exemption.[40] Any value more than this is subtracted from your lifetime estate tax exemption (again, $13.61 in 2024 for single individuals). This means you can give up to $13.61 M in gifts without ever having to pay gift tax. For example, if you gave your child $1M before you died, and then died with $12.61 M, you would owe estate tax on that $1M gift since that gift exceeded the $17,000 limit (meaning it is subtracted from your lifetime gift exemption) and your "net" estate value was $13.61 M. However, if after giving this gift, you died with less than $12.61 M, you would be under the $13.61 M limit and no federal tax would be owed.[41]

Embarking on the path to becoming a successful cardiothoracic surgeon involves many years of education, training, and practice. In doing so, many years are spent perfecting clinical practice, but education in financial well-being is limited. Developing financial literacy is an essential adjunct to clinical education in order to be successful, clinically and personally. Specifically, looking for opportunities to improve financial wellness and developing asset protection is critical for every thoracic surgeon.

DISCLOSURE

The authors have nothing to disclose.

REFERENCES

1. de Brey C. Digest of Education Statistics: 2021. National Center for Education Statistics. Available at: https://nces.ed.gov/programs/digest/d21/foreword.asp. [Accessed 6 September 2023].

2. Appleby C. How many people have student loan debt? Best Colleges. 2023. Accessed: September 6, 2023. Available at: https://www.bestcolleges.com/research/how-many-people-have-student-loans/#:~:text=As%20of%202022%2C%2043.5%20million%20Americans%20have%20federal%20student%20loans.,-Note%20Reference&text=The%20average%20increase%20of%20borrowers,was%20approximately%201%20million%20borrowers.&text=Between%202018%20and%202020%2C%20the,43.5%20million%20borrowers%20in%202022.

3. Haverstock E, Helhoski A, Lane R. Student loan debt statistcs: 2023. Nerdwallet. 2023. Available at: https://www.nerdwallet.com/article/loans/student-loans/student-loan-debt. [Accessed 6 September 2023].

4. Powell F, Kerr F. 13 Advantages of federal student loans. U.S. News and World Report. 2021. Available at: https://www.usnews.com/education/best-colleges/paying-for-college/slideshows/10-advantages-of-federal-student-loans. [Accessed 6 September 2023].

5. Hahn A, Tarver J. Student loan debt statistics: average student loan debt. Forbes Advisor 2023. Available at: https://www.forbes.com/advisor/student-loans/average-student-loan-debt-statistics/. [Accessed 6 September 2023].

6. Wood S. Understanding Federal Student Loan Types. U.S. News and World Report. 2023. Available at: https://www.usnews.com/education/blogs/student-loan-ranger/articles/understanding-the-types-of-federal-student-loans-available. [Accessed 29 October 2023].

7. U.S. Department of Education. Wondering how the amount of your federal student aid is determined? Federal Student Aid. Available at: https://studentaid.gov/complete-aid-process/how-calculated. [Accessed 29 October 2023].

8. Historical Rates. Finaid. Available at: https://finaid.org/loans/historicalrates/. [Accessed 29 October 2023].

9. Lustig M. What to know about student loan origination fees. U.S. News and World Report. 2020. Available at: https://www.usnews.com/education/blogs/student-loan-ranger/articles/what-to-know-about-student-loan-origination-fees. [Accessed 29 October 2023].

10. U.S. Department of Education. (General-23-37) FY 24 Sequester-Required Changes to the Title IV Student Aid Programs, . Federal student aid. Available at: https://fsapartners.ed.gov/knowledge-center/library/electronic-announcements/2023-05-15/fy-24-sequester-required-changes-title-iv-student-aid-programs. [Accessed 29 October 2023].

11. U.S. Department of Education. Who's my student loan servicer? Federal Student Aid. Available at: https://studentaid.gov/manage-loans/repayment/servicers. [Accessed 29 October 2023].

12. U.S. Department of Education. Interest Rates and fees for federal student loans. Available at: https://studentaid.gov/understand-aid/types/loans/interest-rates. [Accessed 29 October 2023].

13. Hahn A, Basile C. Best private student loans 2023. Forbes Advisor; 2023. Available at: https://www.forbes.com/advisor/student-loans/best-private-student-loans/. [Accessed 30 November 2023].

14. Luthi B, Wilkins A. Federal vs. private student loans: What's the difference? Bankrate 2023. Available at: https://www.bankrate.com/loans/student-loans/federal-vs-private-student-loans/#what. [Accessed 29 October 2023].

15. McCullers M, Stefanescu I. "Introducing Section 529 Plans into the U.S. Financial Accounts and Enhanced Financial Accounts," FEDS notes. Washington: Board of Governors of the Federal Reserve System; 2015. https://doi.org/10.17016/2380-7172.1673.

16. Kagan J, Battle A, Kvilhaug S. 529 Plan: What is is, How it works, Pros and cons. Investopedia 2023. Available at: https://www.investopedia.com/terms/1/529plan.asp. [Accessed 30 November 2023].

17. Mesirow. 529 plans aren't just for college anymore. Mesirow. Published: March 2023. Available at: https://www.mesirow.com/wealth-knowledge-center/529-plans-arent-just-college-anymore. [Accessed 29 October 2023].

18. U.S. Securities and Exchange Commission. Updated investor bulletin: a introduction to 529 plans. U.S Securities and Exchange Commission; 2023. Available at: https://www.sec.gov/about/reports-publications/investor-publications/introduction-529-plans. [Accessed 29 October 2023].

19. Hanson M. Average cost per credit hour. Education Data Initiative; 2022. Available at: https://educationdata.org/cost-of-a-college-class-or-credit-hour. [Accessed 29 October 2023].

20. Zinn D, Hahn A. How to pay for college: 5 ways to fund your education now. Forbes Advisor; 2022. Available at: https://www.forbes.com/advisor/student-loans/how-to-pay-for-college/. [Accessed 4 November 2023].

21. U.S. Department of Education. Find and apply for as many scholarships as you can – it's free money for college or career school! Federal Student Aid. Available at: https://studentaid.gov/understand-aid/types/scholarships. [Accessed 4 November 2023].

22. U.S. Department of Education. Federal grants are money to help pay for college or career school. Federal student aid. Available at: https://studentaid.gov/understand-aid/types/grants. [Accessed 4 November 2023].

23. U.S. Department of Education. Federal work-study jobs help students earn money to pay for college or career school. Federal Student Aid. Available at: https://studentaid.gov/understand-aid/types/work-study. [Accessed 4 November 2023].

24. Edwards TGA, Lazzara CJ, Nelesen J, et al. SPIVA U.S. Scorecard. In: S&P dow jones indicies. 2022.

Available at: https://www.spglobal.com/spdji/en/documents/spiva/spiva-us-year-end-2022.pdf. [Accessed 21 October 2023] 2022.

25. Forbes Advisor. 403(b) vs. 401(k): Which is better for retirement?. 2023. Available at: https://www.forbes.com/advisor/retirement/403b-vs-401k/. [Accessed 21 October 2023].

26. Internal Revenue Service. Retirement topics – IRA Contribution Limits. 2023. Available at: https://www.irs.gov/retirement-plans/plan-participant-employee/retirement-topics-ira-contribution-limits. [Accessed 21 October 2023].

27. Internal Revenue Service. Amount of Roth IRA contributions that you can make for 2023. 2023. Available at: https://www.irs.gov/retirement-plans/amount-of-roth-ira-contributions-that-you-can-make-for-2023. [Accessed 21 October 2023].

28. Charles Schwab. Are HSAs the new IRAs?. 2023. Available at: https://www.schwab.com/learn/story/are-hsas-new-iras. [Accessed 21 October 2023].

29. Fernando J, Battle A, Costagliola D. What is disability insurance? Definition and how it protects you. Investopedia 2021. Available at: https://www.investopedia.com/terms/d/disability-insurance.asp. [Accessed 4 November 2023].

30. Hurst A, Swartz A. Elimination periods in disability insurance. Policy Genius 2023. Available at: https://www.policygenius.com/disability-insurance/disability-insurance-elimination-periods/. [Accessed 30 November 2023].

31. Fraraccio M. Short-term vs. long-term disability: what's the difference? U.S. Chamber of Commerce. 2022. Available at: https://www.uschamber.com/co/run/finance/short-term-vs-long-term-disability. [Accessed 4 November 2023].

32. Hurst A, Swartz A. Disability insurance riders. Policy Genius 2023. Available at: https://www.policygenius.com/disability-insurance/what-disability-riders-do-you-need/. [Accessed 4 November 2023].

33. Fontinelle A, Battle A. Life insurance: what it is, how it works, and how to buy a policy. Investopedia. 2023.

Available at: https://www.investopedia.com/terms/l/lifeinsurance.asp. [Accessed 4 November 2023].

34. Term life vs. whole life insurance: differences and how to choose. Nerdwallet. Available at: https://www.nerdwallet.com/l/life-insurance-dyn-3?utm_source=goog&utm_medium=cpc&utm_campaign=li_mktg_paid_082523_dsa&utm_term=&utm_content=ta&mktg_place=dsa-2186806805491&gad=1&gclid=CjwKCAjwpJ-WoBhA8EiwAHZFzfiWq_D_DfsjgOPQ0MC2pIxxfVOKx0-HkgElKmBhmQeU7qTjSWNFJ2KRoCddkQAvD_BwE&gclsrc=aw.ds. [Accessed 4 November 2023].

35. Schlichter S, Constantine C, Cude BJ. What is umbrella insurance, and how does it work? Nerdwallet. 2023. Available at: https://www.nerdwallet.com/article/insurance/umbrella-insurance. [Accessed 30 November 2023].

36. Kagan J. Revocable Trust Definition. Investopedia 2022.

37. Kagan J. Pour-Over Will Definition and How it Works with a Trust. Investopedia 2023. Available at: https://www.investopedia.com/terms/p/pour-overwill.asp. [Accessed 1 November 2023].

38. Internal Revenue Service. Estate and gift taxes. 2023. Available at: https://www.irs.gov/businesses/small-businesses-self-employed/estate-and-gift-taxes. [Accessed 1 November 2023].

39. Morgan JP. New York Estate Planning. 2023. Available at: https://www.jpmorgan.com/insights/wealth-planning/estate-planning/new-york-estate-planning#:~:text=Generally%2C%20for%20New%20York%20-estate,estate%20taxes%20will%20be%20due. [Accessed 20 October 2023].

40. Schwab Charles. The Estate tax and Lifetime Gifting. 2023. Available at: https://www.schwab.com/learn/story/estate-tax-and-lifetime-gifting. [Accessed 20 October 2023].

41. Federal income tax rates and brackets. 2023. Available at: https://www.irs.gov/filing/federal-income-tax-rates-and-brackets.

Hobbies, Distractions, Obsessions, and Addictions

Shubham Gulati, MS[a,b,1],*, M. Blair Marshall, MD[c]

KEYWORDS

- Work-life balance • Well-being • Lifestyle • Outside interests • Cardiothoracic surgery

KEY POINTS

- Hobbies play an essential role in countering the stresses of a career in cardiothoracic (CT) surgery.
- Balancing outside interests with work is critical and necessary to maintain one's well-being and thrive at work and outside of work.
- Inappropriate focus on distractions or obsessions can be detrimental to one's work and patient care and is a sign of underlying problems.
- CT surgeons are at high risk for alcohol and substance abuse and suicidal ideation, a risk factor for suicide.

INTRODUCTION

A discussion of wellness in thoracic surgery necessitates addressing why wellness matters in the first place. Luckily, the answer is obvious. Wellness is necessary for thoracic surgeons to excel at their job, remain committed to the field, and educate the next generation. Our future depends upon it. Physician well-being is necessary for surgeons, and individuals practicing health care in general, to be able to treat their patients and patients' families with the utmost compassion and care at all times. In the field of medicine, we have failed to ensure physician wellness. With many of the current changes in health care, it is no surprise that the modern medical landscape is ripe with discussions of physician dissatisfaction and burnout. Moral injury has become the "vogue" phrase. Physician wellness has become such a critical problem that both the US Surgeon General's office and American Medical Association have made advocating for it a priority.[1,2] Poor well-being and burnout have led many physicians to change careers or retire.[3,4] For some, it has gone beyond just the end or change of one's career. An anonymous survey with nearly 8000 surgeons responding found the degree of burnout experienced was independently associated with suicidal ideation, while controlling for personal and professional characteristics.[5] This is concerning as suicidal ideation is a risk factor for suicide attempts and suicide is a disproportionate cause of mortality in physicians compared to individuals in other careers and the general population.[6–8] Clearly we have a problem and there is a drastic need for improved well-being among physicians.[9]

The prevalence of burnout among physicians has increased over recent decades. The coronavirus disease 2019 pandemic fostered our realization of this dire situation.[10] Thoracic surgeons are not immune from these effects. To increase awareness, a recent survey was published from

[a] Icahn School of Medicine at Mount Sinai, Mount Sinai Health System, New York, NY, USA; [b] Division of Thoracic Surgery, Brigham and Women's Hospital, Harvard Medical School, Boston, MA, USA; [c] Division of Thoracic Surgery, Sarasota Memorial Hospital, Sarasota, FL, USA
[1] Present address: 504 Northwest 154th Street, Edmond, OK 73013.
* Corresponding author. Icahn School of Medicine at Mount Sinai, One Gustave L. Levy Place, Box 1255, New York, NY 10029.
E-mail address: shubham.gulati@icahn.mssm.edu

Thorac Surg Clin 34 (2024) 233–238
https://doi.org/10.1016/j.thorsurg.2024.04.002
1547-4127/24/© 2024 Elsevier Inc. All rights reserved.

the Wellness Committee of the American Association for Thoracic Surgery (AATS). Seventy percent of survey respondents felt that burnout affected their personal relationships at times and 43% experienced a great deal of work-related stress.[11]

Thoracic surgeons are often drawn to the stress of our profession, finding professional satisfaction in being able to provide solutions for some of the most challenging clinical situations. If so, then why are thoracic surgeons experiencing burnout? In part, it is due to the fact that the difficulty of a career in thoracic surgery bleeds into activities that can relieve the stress of our vocation. In a survey of significant others of cardiothoracic (CT) surgeons, the AATS Wellness Committee found that 63% of respondents found their partner's work load did not leave enough time for family.[12] 58% reported that their CT surgeon partner had less connection with outside interests and hobbies. These factors contribute to burnout and should be addressed directly. Analysis of US surgeon burnout showed that collegial support for work-life integration was independently associated with career satisfaction and insufficient time for family was independently associated with lower career satisfaction.[13]

From experience, the rise in burnout among surgeons and physicians may be in part a result of the changing health care environment. As a whole, the practice of medicine has shifted from several decades ago. Physicians were more autonomous and felt valued by the hospital in which they worked. The more recent model as hospital employee has led to the erosion of autonomy and feelings that one is just a gear in the machine of health care. There is constant pressure to generate relative value units.[14] With this, can one have true equipoise when deciding whether or not to operate? In addition, physicians are forced to balance patient care with cost containment and additional pressures from hospital administration. More and more nonclinical tasks are assigned. And on top of that are the reviews of performance by both internet surveys and random metrics that seem not to truly evaluate the quality of care. For many surgeons, the added pressure of balancing clinical responsibilities and best care with academic and research productivity in addition to education and mentorship can be just overwhelming. Despite the increasing responsibilities and expectations for physicians, the amount of time in the day remains constant. Documentation requirements, regulatory compliance trainings, administrative meetings, and more continue to eat away at our time, pulling us away from what drew us to the field.

With a changing practice, some struggle to find why we chose a career as a CT surgeon in the mire that consumes much of our work today. Those who have successfully completed the preparation and training required to be a CT surgeon have likely become used to a level of achievement and success. Our field is one that draws individuals driven to excel, whether that be in patient care, academic research, technical skills, or innovative endeavors. Yet, the components we trained ourselves to excel at, surgery and patient care, may no longer consume the majority of our day. Although these additional requirements are often necessary to function in our health system, they leave us feeling empty, lacking the satisfaction and gratification we previously drew from the true practice of CT surgery.

The patients and pathology we see and treat have changed as well, often increasing in complexity. There is no denying that CT surgery today is not what it once was. Less than 100 years ago, Dr Evarts A. Graham performed the first 1-stage pneumonectomy for lung cancer, revolutionizing the approach to treating this malignancy.[15] With current advances, today, a thoracic surgeon is regularly able to provide curative surgery to early-stage lung cancer patients. But, today's patients are older and regularly present with multiple comorbidities, making operations more difficult and the risk of complications more likely. A similar story holds for cardiac surgery, with advanced technologies and procedures allowing one to offer lifesaving procedures to patients who would have never previously survived. It is certainly wonderful to have the opportunity to take part in the continuation of a patients' life, but the stress of increased surgical risk of morbidity and mortality is likely underrecognized. These complexities add to the already-immense stress experienced by CT surgeons, contributing to the toll on one's well-being.

As a whole, this issue of *Thoracic Surgery Clinics* provides a well-needed discussion of the many factors affecting CT surgeon well-being, and this article seeks to focus on the importance of balancing work and life outside of work. If we hope to retain people in the practice of thoracic surgery, we must appreciate that we should maintain interests outside of the hospital. Times have changed. The intensity of work in the past does not reflect the work today, with all of its additional stresses. In a field where discussions of work-life balance were historically taboo, it is important to reflect on and understand the potential role and impact of hobbies, distractions, obsessions, and addictions.

Hobbies take us out of the hospital, giving us the chance to interact with others and explore a niche outside of our area of expertise. It should not come as a surprise that hobbies can improve our well-being. Studies have demonstrated that enjoyable leisure activities are associated with higher positive psychosocial states, lower levels of depression and negative affect, and improved physiologic measures.[16] The benefit hobbies provide has been published in the field of medicine as well. Making time for hobbies has been correlated with decreased dysfunction for both orthopedic surgery residents and faculty.[17] Similarly, a survey of Korean surgeons showed that having a hobby reduced occupational stress.[18]

While not rigorously studied in CT surgery, there is no reason the benefits of hobbies would not extend to us. In a field that is inherently difficult and often draining, hobbies can provide respite from the woes of the hospital and patient care, an emotional break. While we, as CT surgeons, have found a love for the work and the impact we make, our journey often also leads us to derive self-worth from the practice of surgery itself. We strive for perfection, aiming for low complication rates and improved patient outcomes. While this goal of perfection is necessary to take the best care of our patients, it takes a psychological toll. Some complications are unavoidable and when they occur, they often have a negative impact on our psyche as we bear the responsibility of provoking the complications. Patient and family response to these events can add to the negative psychological impact and associated stress.

Hobbies provide an outlet, allowing for imperfection and an opportunity to make mistakes. They give us the opportunity to focus on and excel at something completely different from surgery. Based on the type of hobby one pursues, the benefits can be more extensive. As humans, the benefits of exercise and relationships still apply to us.[19,20] Hobbies that incorporate physical activity and promote a sense of community pose additional benefits for CT surgeons.

The idea that hobbies are important for physicians is not novel. One of the founding fathers of modern-day residency programs, Sir William Osler, recognizing that hobbies are essential to counter the stresses of medicine in 1905, wrote, "While medicine is to be your vocation, or calling, see to it that you also have an avocation."[21] While medicine has changed over the past century, Osler's claim that having leisure activities relates to increased engagement in medicine was put to the test in 2011 by McManus and colleagues.[22] In this study, nearly 3000 doctors in the United Kingdom were surveyed covering topics of stress, depersonalization (burnout), emotional exhaustion, personal achievement (vocation), work engagement, and 29 different leisure activities (avocation), in addition to several other factors. Their analysis found that, consistent with Osler's claim, independent of a number of other variables, physicians who had avocation/leisure activities were also more likely to have a greater sense of vocation/engagement.[22]

The leaders of our profession have advocated for leisurely pursuits. In Richard E. Clark's 1990 presidential address to the Southern Thoracic Surgical Association, he cited Osler's writing: "No man is really happy or safe without a hobby, and it makes precious little difference what the outside interest may be."[23] This quote was again referred to in another presidential lecture of the Southern Thoracic Surgical Association again, followed by the statement that "a complete cardiothoracic surgeon should have a hobby outside of medicine. [...] There is something that each of us needs: a diversion outside of the laboratory and operating theater."[24] Most recently, in his presidential addresses at the 2023 World Conference on Lung Cancer, Paul van Schil, a thoracic surgeon, discussed his role as a tour guide at his local zoo.[25]

The research backs it and leaders in the field of medicine and of thoracic surgery harp on it, then why have we, as a field, not come to realize that support systems must exist to encourage a balance between work and life outside of work.

While the process of identifying a hobby is outside the scope of this article, it is important to acknowledge that CT surgeons across the world have found ways to maintain a variety of hobbies. From public activities, like being a tour guide at a zoo, to private activities, like woodworking, CT surgeons have found countless ways to engage in their passions outside of work and balance the stresses of surgery. With any leisure activity you can think of, there is most likely a CT surgeon that has a found a way to balance it with their practice.

However, the need to maintain an "avocation" must not become an additional stressor. We must not create an unyielding image of a perfect CT surgeon as one who is able to manage a hobby along with a bustling surgical practice and strong academic laboratory. In a field of perfectionists, it is expectations like this that can cause more harm than benefit. Our goal must simply remain to encourage and support our colleagues to maintain interests outside of work, identify ways of relieving stress, and pursue their nonacademic/external passions, ensuring personal well-being is prioritized.

We would be amiss if we only addressed the positives of exploring activities outside of work. As with anything, hobbies exist on a spectrum. The engagement of a leisurely pursuit provides a needed distraction from our profession and professional environment. Too much time dedicated to a hobby and it can transform into a detrimental distraction, even an obsession. Although we are all different, and the reasons for choosing this career are varied, on some level, we are all good at focusing. The effort it takes to prepare for this vocation requires a tenacity that can border on obsession. This underlying ability or tendency that we all in part have, when out of control, can lead to obsessive behaviors. While maintaining life outside of the workplace is necessary for well-being, as with many things, balance is needed.

In dealing with the stresses of our work, often including the stresses of family and life in general, like everyone, surgeons seek coping mechanisms. Alcohol is readily accessible, socially acceptable, and for some, provides respite from the stress impacting our wellness. However, this and other substances are addictive. Repeatedly relying on these as a means of escape often becomes substance abuse. While the incidence of alcohol abuse and dependence in the adult population is 11.3%, the incidence in surgeons is higher.[26] In a study conducted by Oreskovich and colleagues, 15.4% of surgeons had a score consistent with alcohol abuse or dependence on the Alcohol Use Disorder Identification Test. This was strongly associated with emotional exhaustion and depersonalization domains of burnout. Staggeringly, among female surgeons, 25.6% had scores consistent with alcohol abuse or dependence.[27]

Carrie Cunningham, likely one of the most accomplished endocrine surgeons in the country, addressed this topic by revealing her recent battle with alcohol addiction during her presidential address for the 2023 Association for Academic Surgery.[28] It was through rehabilitation programs and the support of her colleagues that she was able to recover from her addiction and continue her role as section head of the endocrine surgery program at Massachusetts General Hospital. Her story highlights the difficulties of handling life as a surgeon and draws attention to the consequences when we fail at physician well-being. Dr Cunningham has continued to use her platform to increase awareness of physician depression and for improving mental health practices in our field.[29]

Importantly, with suicidal ideation in 1 of 10 surgeons, entering the profession itself becomes a risk factor for suicide, along with depression and addiction.[30,31] This issue of *Thoracic Surgery Clinics* is critical. For those who are challenged, surgeons should know there are means of obtaining help. Individuals can volunteer for a professional evaluation by state-specific groups such as Massachusetts Medical Society's Physician Health Services and the New York Committee for Physician Health, among others.[32,33] Programs like these provide confidential consultation and support specifically for physicians, residents, and medical students struggling with substance use, mental health, and behavioral health problems. However, medical licensing applications and employment and credentialing applications all include questions about previous diagnosis of mental illness of substance abuse disorder. This is an enormous deterrent to physicians when considering seeking need for help. Knowing this, we must acknowledge that it is very likely that surgeons will not reach out for help. By the numbers, we have an epidemic of mental health issues in our profession. Recognizing this, we all must know or work with someone who is not succeeding in managing their mental health. As a specialty, we must ensure we recognize the signs and provide support for our colleagues who may be struggling.

CT surgery is an extremely difficult field. An average day is focused on treating very sick patients with complicated pathology using skills that require years of training and experience to master. If that were all we needed to do to be successful, it would be much easier. The changes in the health care environment contribute significantly to our stress and sense of moral injury. It is critical to recognize that maintaining our own well-being is a priority and requires effort. Hobbies clearly play a role in this, and it is important for all surgeons to find passions outside of the operating room. Luckily this can look like anything from gardening, to playing sports, to finding ways to engage with family and friends. There are so many activities one can focus some effort on outside of work, and these all vary in the amount of time they require. Regardless of the activity, it is clear that leisure activities play a critical role in our well-being and career engagement. However, not everyone will be successful. We must acknowledge that while striving to find ways to cope with the difficulties of our work, some will lose control. Beyond maintaining our own well-being, we must be on the lookout for those who may not be succeeding in their own wellness. When hobbies progress to becoming detrimental distractions, obsessions, or even addictions, we must address the threat this is to us and our patients and seek support. If we hope to address burnout and addiction, we, CT surgeons, must embrace and encourage discussions of and pursuits of well-being. We must walk the walk not just talk the talk and promote wellness by demonstrating our commitment to wellness in ourselves and among our colleagues.

DISCLOSURE

Dr M.B. Marshall has received honoraria and grant funding from Intuitive Surgical, Inc. United States, and honoraria from Siemens Inc, Germany. The other authors report no conflicts of interest.

REFERENCES

1. Health worker burnout — current priorities of the U.S. surgeon general. Available at: https://www.hhs.gov/surgeongeneral/priorities/health-worker-burnout/index.html. [Accessed 28 November 2023].
2. AMA Recovery plan for america's physicians: reducing physician burnout. American Medical Association. Available at: https://www.ama-assn.org/amaone/ama-recovery-plan-america-s-physicians-reducing-physician-burnout. [Accessed 28 November 2023].
3. Shanafelt TD, Dyrbye LN, West CP, et al. Career plans of US physicians after the first 2 years of the COVID-19 pandemic. Mayo Clin Proc 2023;98(11):1629–40.
4. Rotenstein LS, Brown R, Sinsky C, et al. The association of work overload with burnout and intent to leave the job across the healthcare workforce during COVID-19. J Gen Intern Med 2023;38(8):1920–7.
5. Shanafelt TD, Balch CM, Dyrbye L, et al. Special report: suicidal ideation among American surgeons. Arch Surg 2011;146(1):54–62.
6. Kalmoe MC, Chapman MB, Gold JA, et al. Physician suicide: a call to action. Mo Med 2019;116(3):211.
7. Schernhammer ES, Colditz GA. Suicide rates among physicians: a quantitative and gender assessment (meta-analysis). Am J Psychiatry 2004;161(12):2295–302.
8. Center C, Davis M, Detre T, et al. Confronting depression and suicide in physicians: a consensus statement. JAMA 2003;289(23):3161–6.
9. Burnout is a health crisis for doctors—and patients. American Medical Association; 2023. Available at: https://www.ama-assn.org/about/leadership/burnout-health-crisis-doctors-and-patients. [Accessed 28 November 2023].
10. Shanafelt TD, West CP, Dyrbye LN, et al. Changes in burnout and satisfaction with work-life integration in physicians during the first 2 years of the COVID-19 pandemic. Mayo Clin Proc 2022;97(12):2248–58.
11. Bremner RM, Ungerleider RM, Ungerleider J, et al. Well-being of cardiothoracic surgeons in the time of COVID-19: a survey by the wellness committee of the american association for thoracic surgery.

Semin Thorac Cardiovasc Surg 2022;S1043-0679(22):00254. Published online October 14.
12. Ungerleider JD, Ungerleider RM, James L, et al. Assessment of the well-being of significant others of cardiothoracic surgeons. J Thorac Cardiovasc Surg 2023;S0022-5223(23):00331–8. Published online May 7.
13. Johnson HM, Irish W, Strassle PD, et al. Associations between career satisfaction, personal life factors, and work-life integration practices among US surgeons by gender. JAMA Surg 2020;155(8):742–50.
14. Ikonomidis JS, Boden N, Atluri P. STS thoracic surgery practice and access task force - 2019 workforce report. Ann Thorac Surg 2020;110(3):1082–90.
15. Khaitan PG, D'Amico TA. Milestones in thoracic surgery. J Thorac Cardiovasc Surg 2018;155(6):2779–89.
16. Pressman SD, Matthews KA, Cohen S, et al. Association of enjoyable leisure activities with psychological and physical well-being. Psychosom Med 2009;71(7):725–32.
17. Sargent MC, Sotile W, Sotile MO, et al. Quality of life during orthopaedic training and academic practice. Part 1: orthopaedic surgery residents and faculty. J Bone Joint Surg Am 2009;91(10):2395–405.
18. Kang SH, Boo YJ, Lee JS, et al. High occupational stress and low career satisfaction of Korean surgeons. J Korean Med Sci 2015;30(2):133–9.
19. Thompson WR, Sallis R, Joy E, et al. Exercise is medicine. Am J Lifestyle Med 2020;14(5):511–23.
20. Martino J, Pegg J, Frates EP. The connection prescription: using the power of social interactions and the deep desire for connectedness to empower health and wellness. Am J Lifestyle Med 2015;11(6):466–75.
21. Osler W. Aequanimitas. 3rd edition. London: H K Lewis; 1932.
22. McManus IC, Jonvik H, Richards P, et al. Vocation and avocation: leisure activities correlate with professional engagement, but not burnout, in a cross-sectional survey of UK doctors. BMC Med 2011;9:100.
23. Clark RE. Who, hobbies, and heroes. Ann Thorac Surg 1990;49(4):515–21.
24. Miller JI. The complete cardiothoracic surgeon: qualities of excellence. Ann Thorac Surg 2004;78(1):2–8.
25. Van Schil P. Incoming President's Address. Oral presentation presented at: world conference on lung cancer; 2023; Singapore.
26. Alcohol use disorder (AUD) in the United States: age groups and demographic characteristics | national institute on alcohol abuse and alcoholism (NIAAA). Available at: https://www.niaaa.nih.gov/alcohols-effects-health/alcohol-topics/alcohol-facts-and-statistics/alcohol-use-disorder-aud-united-states-

age-groups-and-demographic-characteristics. [Accessed 28 November 2023].

27. Oreskovich MR, Kaups KL, Balch CM, et al. Prevalence of alcohol use disorders among American surgeons. Arch Surg 2012;147(2):168–74.

28. Cunningham C. AAS Presidential Address - Removing the Mask. Oral Presentation presented at: February 8, 2023. 2023. Available at: https://www.academicsurgicalcongress.org/.

29. Frangou C. US surgeons are killing themselves at an alarming rate. One decided to speak out. Guardian 2023. Available at: https://www.theguardian.com/us-news/2023/sep/26/surgeons-suicide-doctors-physicians-mental-health. [Accessed 28 November 2023].

30. A tragedy of the profession: medscape physician suicide report. Medscape 2022. Available at: https://www.medscape.com/slideshow/2022-physician-suicide-report-6014970. [Accessed 28 November 2023].

31. Menon NK, Shanafelt TD, Sinsky CA, et al. Association of physician burnout with suicidal ideation and medical errors. JAMA Netw Open 2020;3(12): e2028780. https://doi.org/10.1001/jamanetworkopen.2020.28780.

32. Physician health services. Available at: https://www.massmed.org/phshome/. [Accessed 28 November 2023].

33. New york committee for physician health. Available at: https://www.fsphp.org/new-york. [Accessed 28 November 2023].

Abuse, Bullying, Harassment, Discrimination, and Allyship in Cardiothoracic Surgery

Nicolas Contreras, MD[a], Rachael Essig, MD[b], Jessica Magarinos, MD[c], Sara Pereira, MD[d],*

KEYWORDS

- Abuse • Bullying • Harassment • Discrimination • Allyship • Cardiothoracic surgery
- Diversity and inclusion

KEY POINTS

- Abuse, bullying, harassment, and discrimination are issues prominent in surgical specialties that cause burnout and threaten surgeon wellness.
- The cardiothoracic (CT) surgery workforce must prioritize mentorship, sponsorship, and allyship to promote a diverse and healthy specialty for CT surgeon recruitment, growth, and job satisfaction.
- CT surgery and institutional leadership must address and eliminate abuse, bullying, harassment, and discrimination to create a culture of inclusion in our specialty.

INTRODUCTION

Well-being in cardiothoracic (CT) surgery has become an increasingly common area of research and academic focus. It is no longer a secret that burnout and lack of workplace satisfaction are prevalent not only within our specialty but also within our training programs. In a 2020 Thoracic Surgery Residency Association (TSRA) survey, 75% of thoracic surgery trainees indicated that training had a negative impact on their personal relationships, while greater than 50% indicated training negatively impacted their health. While the response rate of the survey was only 20%, greater than 50% of trainees who completed the survey were dissatisfied with their work-life balance. Nearly 50% of respondents screened positive for depression or burnout, and greater than 25% would not enter and complete CT surgery training again.[1] These responses are alarming, and it is easy to assume that the lack of well-being of CT surgery trainees is a function of their intense training circumstances that allow little time for self-care and prioritization of well-being.

Alarmingly, parallel trends are observed in the active CT surgeon workforce. In a recent American Association of Thoracic Surgery (AATS) Wellness Committee survey looking at wellness and burnout during the coronavirus disease 2019 (COVID) pandemic, 50% of practicing CT surgeons reported a sense of "dread" coming to work, half reported a sense of physical or emotional exhaustion at work, 44% reported they seldom or never had adequate time to spend with family, and 52% of

[a] Division of Cardiothoracic Surgery, University of Utah and Huntsman Cancer Institute, 1950 Circle of Hope Drive, Salt Lake City, UT 84112, USA; [b] Department of Surgery, Georgetown University Hospital, 3800 Reservoir Road, PHC4, Washington, DC 20007, USA; [c] Department of Surgery, Temple University, 3401 North Broad Street, Philadelphia, PA 19147, USA; [d] Division of Cardiothoracic Surgery, Department of Surgery, University of Utah, 30 North Mario Capecchi Drive, 4N133, Salt Lake City, UT 84112, USA
* Corresponding author.
E-mail address: Sara.pereira@hsc.utah.edu
Twitter: @RachaelEssig (R.E.); @saraj_pereira (S.P.)

Thorac Surg Clin 34 (2024) 239–247
https://doi.org/10.1016/j.thorsurg.2024.04.001
1547-4127/24/© 2024 Elsevier Inc. All rights reserved.

respondents felt burnout had an impact on their care of patients. Several of respondents (70%) reported that burnout affected their personal relationships at least "some of the time" and 62% noted that they have only scarce or no resources at their institution to provide emotional support to themselves or to a partner. Most respondents (57%) felt that the COVID pandemic negatively affected their well-being. While the survey reports a somewhat encouragingly figure that 63% of CT surgeons reported to "agree" or "strongly agree" that they were satisfied with their job, and 76% were likely to pursue a career in CT surgery again, if given the opportunity, this leaves a sobering 24% to 37% of surgeons who are equivocal about their work satisfaction and desire to pursue the specialty again.[2]

When faced with such overwhelming dissatisfaction affecting both CT surgery trainees and active CT surgeons, it is imperative to assess the potential workplace barriers that exist for surgeon well-being in our specialty: chiefly, the presence of abuse, bullying, harassment, and discrimination. While well-being is known to include much more than just the absence of an abusive workplace environment, surgeon well-being cannot begin to flourish with these factors actively present and commonly reported in the workplace. Furthermore, and equally as important, the presence of allyship in the CT surgery workplace needs to be encouraged with increasing diversification of our specialty in recent years. In this article, we desire to explore these prevalent barriers to workplace well-being - abuse, bullying, harassment, discrimination - and the presence of allyship in CT Surgery.[3–6]

BACKGROUND
Current Demographics of Cardiothoracic Surgery

As a surgical community looking to make strides toward embracing inclusion, diversity and workplace well-being, the knowledge of the racial, ethnic and gender landscape of CT surgery is an essential stepping-stone. The barriers to workplace wellness (ie, abuse, bullying, harassment, and discrimination), are all accentuated by the power differentials between different groups in the workplace. Knowledge about the racial, ethnic, and gender makeup of our community becomes a critical component of work wellness dialogues. At baseline, it is important to note that the metric "lens" through which diversity in CT surgery should be measured by is via a comparison to the diversity present within the US population - the population that CT surgeons strive to serve.[7]

In other words, the diversity breakdown present in the US population should be the diversity breakdown that exists within members of the CT surgery workforce. Those racial or ethnic groups that have representation in medicine below that of the general population are classified as Underrepresented in Medicine (URiM) (**Table 1**).[3–6]

By 2020 US Census Data, 50.4% of citizens identified as women. Non-Hispanic Whites made up 58.9% of the population. Hispanics and Latinos comprised 19.1%, Blacks or African Americans 13.6%, Asians 6.3%, American Indians 1.3%, and Pacific Islanders or Native Hawaiians 0.3%.[8] Within CT surgery training programs in 2019, several of the CT trainees identified as White (58%), with the remainder identifying as Asian (18%), Hispanic (4%), and Black (3%).[9] Similar trends are seen at the academic faculty level with 63% of CT surgery faculty identifying as White, 24% Asian American, 5% Hispanic, and 3% Black.[10] Significant advancements have been made in improving gender equality in medicine as a whole, as currently half of all medical school graduates are women. Even in surgical subspecialties such as General Surgery, 46% of surgical trainees are women. This positive trend has unfortunately not carried into CT surgery. In 2019, only 24% of CT trainees identified as women.[9,11] At higher professional levels, women comprise less than 20% of CT academic faculty.[11] Despite the increasing trend of women in medicine

Table 1	
Definitions of underrepresented in medicine, mentorship, sponsorship, and allyship	
	Definition
Underrepresented in Medicine	Racial and ethnic populations that are underrepresented in the medical profession relative to their numbers in the general population[3]
Mentorship	The influence, guidance, or direction given by a mentor[4]
Sponsorship	One who assumes responsibility for some other person or thing[5]
Allyship	Supportive association with another group, specifically members of a marginalized or mistreated groups to which one does not belong[6]

and as trainees, CT surgery remains one of the least diverse specialties in medicine and surgery.[12]

It is important to acknowledge the critical elements that a diverse workforce brings to a healthy working environment. Workplace injustices or "barriers to well-being" (ie, abuse, bullying, harassment, and discrimination) are more likely to be experienced by minority groups than demographic majority groups. These workplace injustices are linked to poor psychological and health outcomes, as well as poor work-related outcomes.[13] It subsequently follows that the agenda to achieve workplace well-being must be intimately associated with an effort to achieve a diverse and inclusive workforce. One cannot succeed without the other. It is not just the physician workforce who benefits from this initiative. Patient and hospital-related outcomes additionally improve when care is delivered by a more diverse workforce.[14]

Abuse in Cardiothoracic Surgery

While there is considerable overlap in definitions amongst abuse, bullying, harassment, and discrimination, there are subtle differences. They all represent forms of workplace injustice and are known to contribute to physician burnout in medicine and surgery. Burnout represents a syndrome of emotional exhaustion, cynicism, depersonalization, and reduced effectiveness at work, and has been attributed to increased medical errors, depression, and physician suicide.[15] The prevalence of burnout is highest amongst surgeons, trainees, and women than in other groups and places physicians at risk for leaving medicine, substance abuse, and suicidal ideation.[16,17] This phenomenon is not isolated from CT surgery as roughly half of CT surgeons experience burnout throughout their training or career.[1,2]

Abuse is any action or failure to act that causes intentional or unintentional suffering and harm to a person. It can be characterized by verbal, emotional, or physical forms. While the incidence of abusive behavior in the CT community has not been as readily studied as in other specialties, trends in other surgical subspecialties can be used to infer the likely incidence within CT surgery. In a comprehensive national survey administered to 99% of general surgery residents in US training programs, verbal or emotional abuse was reported by 30.2% of all residents, 33% of women, and 28.2% of men. Sources of abusive behaviors were attending surgeons (55.2%) and other residents (20.2%), while physical abuse was only rarely reported (2.2%). Individuals who experienced regular abuse were at much higher risk of reporting burnout (odds ratio 2.94) and suicidal ideation (odds ratio 3.07).[15] Given these higher rates of career dissatisfaction and burnout amongst CT surgeons compared with other surgical specialties, a more focused effort needs to take place studying the forms of abuse experienced by CT surgeons during training and active practice.[18,19] As CT surgery is a surgical specialty that remains unique amongst others because of the prolonged training requirements and work-hours, it requires more focused studies analyzing the elements that lead to abuse and toxic work environments. For example, in other non-medical work environments, the lack of inclusivity has been reported as one of the top contributors to a toxic work culture and a leading reason for dissatisfaction and turnover.[20] In order to effectively address issues with burnout and abuse, we need to better understand factors that contribute to current environmental and cultures.

BULLYING AND HARASSMENT IN CARDIOTHORACIC SURGERY

Bullying and harassment are forms of abuse and workplace mistreatment. They represent more specific and potentially more harmful subtypes of abuse. Bullying is a subcategory of harassment and entails a repetitive pattern of aggressive behavior between 2 persons holding imbalanced positions of power.[21] Interestingly, the target of bullying may not realize that they are experiencing bullying for a period of time. Harassment, in contrast, is a serious offense that involves unwanted behavior that humiliates, offends, or intimidates another person and is often obvious to the victim from its onset. Both bullying and harassment involve undesired words and actions toward another person that victimizes one individual over another. The incidence of both bullying and harassment in CT communities has been documented in the US, as well as abroad. A survey administered across surgical specialties in Australia indicated that 49% of responding CT surgeons have experienced bullying in the workplace.[22] This was the highest of all surgical subspecialties surveyed. Bullying and harassment tend to be more prevalent in workplace structures where substantial hierarchies are present, such as in surgery and CT surgery. Additionally, the enduring rigid and tough surgical traditions and teaching styles still present in academic hospitals despite elimination of pyramidal training programs allow for bullying and harassment to linger and sometimes remain many times unchallenged and accepted as the norm.[23,24] And just as in abuse, the presence of bullying and harassment has substantial implications on physician well-being and burnout.[25]

While harassment represents a large multifaceted topic, specific types of harassment have been frequently outlined in the medical literature and represent complex categories: gender-based harassment and racial/ethnic harassment.

Gender-Based Harassment

For decades there have been reports of gender-based harassment during surgical training and beyond. In the 1990s, harassment was reported to be significantly higher for women trainees compared with male in both General Surgery and CT training programs.[26] Types of gender-based harassment include microaggressions, being mistaken for a non-physician, and hurtful uncomfortable slurs and comments. Acts of sexual harassment can range from explicit crude comments, unwanted verbal sexual attention, unwanted physical proximity, and sexual coercion. Both gender-based and sexual harassment can be perpetrated by direct supervisors, work colleagues, patients, and nursing staff.[27–29] Victims of sexual harassment can experience several different sequalae after being victimized including post-traumatic stress disorder and suicidal ideation. Of attending CT surgeons, 81% of female surgeons experienced sexual harassment and 19% reported being victims of sexual coercion.[30] Direct reporting and institutional action occur in only a small number of cases because of fear of retribution and belief that reporting will not change action or outcome. In a survey to surgery, anesthesia, and medicine residents at 2 large academic institutions, an overwhelming majority of both men (86%) and women (96%) respondents either experienced or observed gender-biased discrimination in the training environment. Less than 5% of respondents formally reported such experiences, most frequently citing a belief that nothing would happen.[27,28]

While women are more likely to be victims of gender-based and sexual harassment, men are not excluded from being victims of both types of harassment as well. There are a wide range of reports in the literature, with 17% - 46% of men general and CT surgeons reporting gender-based and sexual harassment. In contrast to women surgeons, however, the perpetrators were more likely to be ancillary staff or physician colleagues. For women, supervising leaders and colleagues are the predominant offenders.[28–31] Additionally, concerning to these statistics, 71% of women and 51% of men CT surgeons have witnessed sexual harassment in the workplace. Only about half of

these individuals reported intervening on the incident when witnessing an event. More women surgeons warned their colleagues of a particular person's behavior compared with men. These trends are also present among CT surgery trainees. Over 90% of women CT surgical trainees have experienced sexual harassment, as compared with 32% of men.[27]

Racial Harassment

There is a paucity of representation of Latino, Black, and Native American physicians and surgeons in the medical community. CT surgery is no different.[10,11,32] Only 3% of surgeons in academic CT practice are Black and only 4% are Latino.[10,11] These figures are alarming when considering the general US population has a racial makeup nearly 4 to 5 times greater for each group, at 13.6% and 19.1%, respectively.[8] Trainees of under-represented ethnic and racial backgrounds commonly feel as if they do not belong in their institution and are uncomfortable to ask for assistance with depression, suicidal ideation, and burnout.[32] Microaggressions are rooted in implicit bias around the expected roles of marginalized groups within healthcare and leadership. Microaggressions can be gender, ethnic, or racially-based and can create negative psychologic side effects with continued exposures. Microaggressions can be micro-invalidations, micro-insults, and micro-assaults. All these can be classified as forms of racial prejudice.[33] While these aggressions may not be as extreme as overt acts of racism, microaggressions may cement feelings of humiliation, intimidation, and lack of belonging, which all cause harm and create a toxic work environment. It has been shown that Black surgical residents are significantly more likely to experience daily microaggressions compared with White surgical residents. Microaggressions further perpetuate the archaic surgical and institutional power hierarchy structures.[32]

Reducing the incidence of harassment in CT surgery is a substantial challenge. In the hierarchical structure of surgery, the individual affected by the bullying or harassment may not initially recognize these actions and behaviors. Furthermore, if individuals do recognize the behavior as bullying or harassment, many do not know how or when to intervene.[23] The term "psychological safety" was popularized by Dr Amy Edmondson from Harvard Business School. This concept describes that persons have a workplace climate where they are comfortable being themselves and speaking openly. Psychologic safety creates the optimal working environment for new idea development without apprehension of retribution.[34] Safety and open expression are critical for the multidisciplinary approach to CT surgery.

Freedom of ethnic and racial harassment and promotion of a more diverse healthcare workforce can additionally lead for improved health outcomes for underrepresented populations. It has been well demonstrated that patients report increased satisfaction with their healthcare if their provider is of the same ethnicity.[31] This positive patient satisfaction is based on better communication and trust for their providers, which correlated with improved compliance with care and treatment programs.[35] The ability to create an inclusive culture and recognize the specific features of bullying and harassment experienced by physicians of diverse ethnic backgrounds is the key to improving the patient outcomes and work environments for both patients and surgeons. Maintaining a diverse workforce assists in providing equitable healthcare, higher patient satisfaction, and care quality. This requires deliberate institutional efforts and frameworks put forth by institutions to garner diverse trainees and faculty.[10,11,31]

DISCRIMINATION IN CARDIOTHORACIC SURGERY

Discrimination is the unjust or prejudicial treatment of different categories of people, especially on the grounds of ethnicity, age, sex, or disability.[36] This prejudicial treatment can manifest as overt gender or racial bias but can occur with subtle microaggressions and implicit bias as discussed earlier. Similar to bullying and harassment, discrimination may be difficult to prove, as the perpetrator may not realize his or her behaviors and biases. The historically homogenous environment and lack of racial, ethnic, and gender diversity in CT surgery has led to the establishment of unwritten barriers that self-propagate the ongoing lack of diversity of the specialty. The presence of these barriers is self-evident when analyzing the trends of diversity from early medical training to the completion of CT surgery training.

Women now have nearly equal representation in medical school admissions and classes. This trend is now sustained in General Surgery residency programs with 46% of residents identifying as women.[37] However, in the transition from medical school and General Surgery residency to CT surgery fellowships, there is a 22% decrease in women CT surgery fellows. This leaves current gender representation in CT surgery to 24% women. Similar trends in racial and ethnic disparities are also seen, although they begin much earlier in the education process. Black and Hispanic students continue to be underrepresented minorities in higher education, medical school classes, and surgical specialties throughout the US. Thirty nine percent of high school students make up URiM groups. Thirty-three percent of URiM high school student pursue undergraduate studies. Of the students applying to medical school and graduating from medical school, only 15% are URiM.[38,39] CT surgery has less than 10% URiM. Many have outlined the leaky pipeline that creates significant differences in racial representation in CT surgery and other surgical specialties. There are known implicit and explicit biases affecting the matriculation of URiM students into secondary and tertiary level education.[38–41] Other studies have shown implicit bias in grading and letter of recommendations for Black and Hispanic surgery applicants that may impact residency opportunities.[42]

Differences in representation in CT surgery foster gender and racial disparities because of lack of mentorship and representation in authorship, and ultimately impact career advancement. Concomitantly these disparities have also created an environment in which underrepresented trainees disproportionately witness and experience gender-based and sexual harassment and discrimination.[43] A recent survey to European Society of Thoracic Surgery and European Association for Cardiothoracic Surgery members discovered that 67% of women CT surgeons had experienced gender discrimination, with 35% reporting that they had considered leaving the specialty because of their negative experiences. Additionally, 60% of women participants reported not having formal mentorship, and only a small percentage of women had participated in a formal leadership or mentorship program. Women CT surgeons also had lower rates of academic publications and grant submissions.[44]

With women and underrepresented minorities in CT surgery facing leaky pipelines, slower rates of publication and promotion, it is clear that the infrastructure of the CT surgery needs to be addressed. The hope certainly is that by addressing representational disparities in CT surgery, the discrimination that underrepresented groups face will improve. Mentorship, sponsorship, and allyship are absolutely critical for success. Practicing CT surgeons must become mentors, sponsors, allies, and upstanders. There is a need of recruitment, support, and retainship of talented physicians and surgeons into the respective specialty.

ALLYSHIP

Allyship is defined as the actions, behaviors, and practices that leaders take to support, amplify, and advocate with others, especially with individuals who do not belong to the same social identity groups as themselves. Other terms for this concept of "allyship" include "champion" and "upstander". Traditionally an "ally" is a person who is a member of a majority or dominant group who supports and takes a stand against injustices and prejudices directed toward a non-dominant marginalized or mistreated group.[45–47] An ally is someone who uses his or her position of power and privilege to advocate for those in marginalized groups.[48] We advance a broader definition of an ally as anyone can advocate for another, regardless of position. For instance, a resident can be an ally for a faculty member experiencing bias. Many underestimate the power they have to stand up for others. Becoming an ally involves active learning, empathy, commitment to recognizing unconscious bias, consistency, and courage (**Table 2**).

MENTORSHIP, SPONSORSHIP, AND ALLYSHIP IN CARDIOTHORACIC SURGERY

The concepts of mentorship, sponsorship, and allyship are a critically important key to creating this optimal working environment in CT surgery. They are important to early, mid, and late career success, and all represent slightly differing behaviors and actions to promote a surgeon's career path and well-being. Approximately 67% of trainees enter the CT surgical field because of the positive impact of their early mentor.[49,50] While having a mentor that is similar to the mentee is often desired by the mentee, there is a concept referred to as the "the minority tax" in which those underrepresented mentors are saddled with a larger mentoring responsibility.[31,51,52] With the

small proportion of women and URiM surgeons in the CT community, the number of URiM surgeons in leadership positions to engage in mentorship and sponsorship is limited. This recognizes that all surgeons who are in a position to provide mentoring and allyship should do so by evaluating the mentee's needs regardless of their personal background. Discordant mentorship and sponsorship should occur across all surgical subspecialties by senior academic and institutional leaders. Within practicing woman CT surgeons, only 58.2% identified their internal division chief or department chair to be an ally. Sixty-hour percent of women respondents considered at least one woman in their department an ally, whereas 14.9% reported no women colleagues within their division.[50] Education with cross-cultural and implicit bias training is also important for mentors. Behaviors surrounding mentorship, support, and sponsorship are the most frequently reported important characteristics of men and women allies. Disrespect, discrimination, stereotyping, and unconscious bias are most often reported as detrimental characteristics of men allies, with competitiveness and undermining as most frequently reported negative characteristics of women colleagues.[50,52]

The Society of Thoracic Surgery (STS) and AATS have identified the lack of diversity as a pivotal issue within the field of CT surgery and have created numerous working groups and initiatives to help address known issues with surgeon wellness. In 2017, then STS President Dr Richard Prager established a Presidential Task Force on Diversity and Inclusion, which subsequently has maintained a high functioning Workforce on Diversity and Inclusion since 2019. It is vital that the STS

Table 2
How to become an ally in cardiothoracic surgery

Educate	Speak	Act
Read, Listen, and Learn	**Use Your Positive Voice**	**Advocate, Support, Sponsor**
• Listen and seek advice from URiM colleagues	• Actively engage in diversity dialogue and conferences	• Be an Ally and Role Model
• Familiarize yourself with the inequalities and challenges that marginalized groups face in surgery	• Avoid derogatory jokes and controversial language	• Join diversity, equity, and inclusion committees
• Acquaint yourself with terminology of diversity	• Do not justify inappropriate remarks in the workplace	• Actively mentor and support URiM physicians and students
• Acknowledge your own bias and privilege that affects your daily life	• Embrace the role of an "upstander" and "champion" in conversations with individuals who display discriminatory behavior	• Create a culture of inclusion at your institution
• Offer implicit bias training for faculty and trainees	• Discuss and prioritize diversity with leadership	• Nominate and recruit URiM colleagues for promotions and leadership opportunities

strive to not only attract and retain the best and brightest inclusive of sex, ethnic background, and other demographics, but also eliminate systematic and implicit biases that hinder the advancement of diverse groups in CT surgery. Annual STS meetings now include the Vivien T. Thomas invited plenary lecture and symposium, which strive to address practice gaps in diversity and inclusion and provide education and leadership tools on the importance of diversification of our national workforce and organizations.[53] Formal efforts through these professional societies have also sought to identify early career surgeons and provide formal mentoring and leadership programs, as well as scholarship opportunities for academic endeavors.[54] Since the establishment of the STS Looking to the Future Scholarship Program in 2006, 669 scholarships have been awarded to medical students and residents to encourage them to pursue CT surgery. Scholars are assigned a national mentor and attend the STS National Meeting, with a planned informative symposium designed for the mentees. With this program, several of residents (63.4%) matriculated into fellowship and became CT surgeons, while roughly one-third (31%) of medical students have become CT residents and surgeons. Nearly 40% of scholarship awardees are women.[55]

The AATS Wellness Committee was established to address wellness issues within CT surgery and how surgeon wellness can be optimized. With results from the AATS Wellness Committee survey, national organization and institutions are sponsoring increased numbers of webinars, educational sessions, and grand rounds discussing these topics and concerns.[2] Core principles of well-being include progress toward a goal, actions commensurate with experience and mission, interconnectivity with other persons, social relatedness, and acceptance, safety, and autonomy.[56] Implementation of a wellness program and curriculum into CT surgery training programs has been emphasized by the Thoracic Surgery Directors Association (TSDA) and Thoracic Surgery Residents Association (TSRA) in recent years. Fajardo and colleagues proposed a CT surgery Wellness "Checklist" and Wellness policy in concordance with Accredition Council for Graduate Medical Education Well-being requirements in 2020, which outlines the establishment of a local wellness culture and includes resident and faculty education, self-screening tools, and fosters a safe work environment for trainees.[17] Wellness programs should provide access to health care, foster a culture of health maintenance, and offer resources for mental health and psychologic counseling for residents and fellows.

In addition to allyship and wellness, there has been a focus on fostering a more inclusive workplace and training environment that does not tolerate discrimination and offers more acceptance for the concept of work life balance. These initiatives include formal departmental family leave policies, and promoting the need for flexibility in call schedules and childcare commitments. Additionally thoracic fellowship programs have critically appraised their application process in an effort to identify and remove implicit bias from their interview process and create a fair recruitment process. Eisenberg and colleagues identified several areas of unintended bias in their recruitment and interview process, including gendered language, cultural bias, and stereotyping in how candidates were scored. They provide recommendations for standardized interview questions and identification of desired applicant characteristics such as emotional intelligence, grit, resilience, and cultural fit.[57] Factors in residency applicant selection that have historically favored non-URiM students such as American Osteopathic Association induction, applicant photos, and number of manuscripts have also been identified as possible sources of bias for residency selection and recruitment.

SUMMARY

Abuse, bullying, harassment, and discrimination threaten the well-being of CT surgeons and the future of our specialty. Organizational and national efforts to promote positive behaviors and education are warranted. With concerted efforts to address gender and racial disparities, allyship, and wellness, it is our hope that the specialty of CT surgery will lead cultural change and support a diverse CT surgical workforce.

DISCLOSURE

The authors have nothing to disclose.

REFERENCES

1. Chow OS, Sudarshan M, Maxfield MW, et al. National survey of burnout and distress among cardiothoracic surgery trainees. Ann Thorac Surg 2021; 111(6):2066–71.
2. Bremner RM, Ungerleider RM, Ungerleider J, et al. Well-being of Cardiothoracic Surgeons in the Time of COVID-19: A Survey by the Wellness Committee of the American Association for Thoracic Surgery. Semin Thorac Cardiovasc Surg 2022;14. S1043-S0679(22)00254-4.
3. AAMC Definition: AAMC. Available at: https://www.aamc.org/what-we-do/equity-diversity-inclusion/under

represented-in-medicine. [Accessed 28 November 2023].

4. Mentorship: Merriam-Webster. Available at: https://wwww.merriam-webster.com/dictionary/mentorship. [Accessed 28 November 2023].

5. Sponsorship: Merriam-Webster. Available at: https://wwww.merriam-webster.com/dictionary/sponsorship. [Accessed 28 November 2023].

6. Allyship: Merriam-Webster. Available at: https://www.merriam-webster.com/dictionary/allyship. [Accessed 28 November 2023].

7. Smedley BD, Stith AY, Colburn L, et al, Institute of Medicine (US). The right thing to do, the smart thing to do: enhancing diversity in the health Professions: Summary of the symposium on diversity in health Professions in Honor of Herbert W. Nickens, M.D. Washington (DC): National Academies Press (US); 2001. Increasing Racial and Ethnic Diversity Among Physicians: An Intervention to Address Health Disparities? Available at: https://www.ncbi.nlm.nih.gov/books/NBK223632. [Accessed 26 November 2023].

8. US Census Bureau.ND.2022 United States Census. United States Department of Commerce. Available at: https://www.census.gov/quickfacts/fact/table/US/PST045222. [Accessed 26 November 2023].

9. Olive JK, Mansoor S, Simpson K, et al. demographic landscape of cardiothoracic surgeons and residents at United States Training Programs. Ann Thorac Surg 2022;114(1):108–14.

10. Ortmeyer KA, Raman V, Tiko-Okoye C, et al. Women and minorities underrepresented in academic cardiothoracic surgery: it's time for next steps. Ann Thorac Surg 2021;112(4):1349–55.

11. Ortmeyer KA, Raman V, Tiko-Okoye C, et al. Goals, organizational change, advocacy, diversity literacy, and sustainability: A checklist for diversity in cardiothoracic surgery training programs. J Thorac Cardiovasc Surg 2021;162(6):1782–7.

12. Antonoff MB, David EA, Donington JS, et al. Women in thoracic surgery: 30 years of history. Ann Thorac Surg 2016;101(1):399–409.

13. Okechukwu CA, Souza K, Davis KD, et al. Discrimination, harassment, abuse, and bullying in the workplace: contribution of workplace injustice to occupational health disparities. Am J Ind Med 2014;57(5):573–86.

14. Gomez LE, Bernet P. Diversity improves performance and outcomes. J Natl Med Assoc 2019;111(4):383–92.

15. Hu YY, Ellis RJ, Hewitt DB, et al. Discrimination, abuse, harassment, and burnout in surgical residency training. N Engl J Med 2019;381(18):1741–52.

16. Rotenstein LS, Torre M, Ramos MA, et al. Prevalence of burnout amongst physicians: A systematic review. JAMA 2018;320(11):1131–50.

17. Fajardo R, Vaporciyan A, Starnes S, et al. Implementation of wellness into a cardiothoracic training program: A checklist for a wellness policy. J Thorac Cardiovasc Surg 2021;161(6):1979–86.

18. Mata DA, Ramos MA, Bansal N, et al. Prevalence of depression and depressive symptoms among resident physicians: a systematic review and meta-analysis. JAMA 2015;314:2373–83.

19. Balch CM, Shanafelt TD, Sloan JA, et al. Distressandcareer satisfaction among 14 surgical specialties, comparing academic and private practice settings. Ann Surg 2011;254:558–68.

20. Sull D, Sull C, Cipolli W, et al. Why every leader needs to worry about toxic culture. 2022. Available at: https://sloanreview.mit.edu/article/why-every-leader-needs-to-worry-about-toxic-culture/. [Accessed 30 November 2023].

21. Halim U, Riding D. Systematic review of the prevalence, impact and mitigating strategies for bullying, undermining behavior and harassment in the surgical workplace. BJS 2018;105:1390–7.

22. Crebbin W, Campbell G, Hillis DA, et al. Prevalence of bullying, discrimination and sexual harassment in surgery in Australasia. ANZ J Surg 2015;85(12):905–9.

23. Gostlow H, Vega Vega C, Marlow N, et al. Do surgeons react? a retrospective analysis of surgeons' response to harassment of a colleague during simulated operating theatre scenarios. Ann Surg 2018;268(2):277–81.

24. Grillo HC. To impart this art: The development of graduate surgical education in the United States. Surgery 1999;125(1):1–14.

25. Gianakos A, Freischlag J, Mercurio A, et al. Bullying, discrimination, harassment, sexual harassment, and the fear of retaliation during surgical residency training: a systemic review. World J Surg 2022;46:1587–99.

26. Dresler C, Padgett D, Mackinnon S, et al. Experiences of women in cardiothoracic surgery. Arch Surg 1996;131:1128–34.

27. Ceppa DP, Dolejs S, Boden N, et al. Sexual harassment and cardiothoracic surgery: #UsToo? Ann Thorac Surg 2020;109(4):1283–8.

28. McKinley SK, Wang LJ, Gartland RM, et al. "Yes, I'm the Doctor": One Department's Approach to Assessing and Addressing Gender-Based Discrimination in the Modern Medical Training Era. Massachusetts General Hospital Gender Equity Task Force. Acad Med 2019;94(11):1691–8.

29. McKinley SK, Parangi S. Addressing sexual harassment in surgical training. Ann Surg 2020;271(4):614–5.

30. Schlick CJR, Ellis RJ, Etkin CD, et al. Experiences of Gender Discrimination and Sexual Harassment Among Residents in General Surgery Programs Across the US. JAMA Surg 2021;156(10):942–52.

31. Erkmen CP, Ortmeyer K, Pelletier G, et al. An approach to diversity and inclusion in cardiothoracic surgery. Ann Thorac Surg 2021;111(3):747–52.

32. Khubchandani J, Atkinson R, Ortega G, et al. Perceived discrimination among surgical residents at academic medical centers. J Surg Res 2022; 272:79–87.

33. Torres MB, Salles A, Cochran A. Recognizing and reacting to microaggressions in medicine and surgery. JAMA Surg 2019;154(9):868–72.

34. Carnahan, B. How to create a psychologically safe workplace. 2023. Harvard Business School Insights and Advice. Available at: https://www.hbs.edu/recruiting/insights-and-advice/blog/post/how-to-create-a-psychologically-safe-workplace; Accessed November 14, 2023.

35. LaVeist TA, Pierre G. Integrating the 3Ds–social determinants, health disparities, and health-care workforce diversity. Publ Health Rep 2014;129(Suppl 2): 9–14.

36. Oxford University Press. Discrimination. Oxford English dictionary. Available at: https://www.oed.com/search/dictionary/?scope=Entries&q=discrimination. [Accessed 30 November 2023].

37. Kearse LE, Jensen RM, Schmiederer IS, et al. Diversity, equity, and inclusion: a current analysis of general surgery residency programs. Am Surg 2022; 88(3):414–8.

38. Moon MR. Equal means equal: Cardiothoracic surgery in its second century. J Thorac Cardiovasc Surg 2021;161(4):1381–9.

39. AAMC 2023 FACTS: Enrollment, Graduates, and MD Data (Tables B-3 and B-4). Available at: https://www.aamc.org/data-reports. [Accessed 30 November 2023].

40. Capers Q, Clinchot D, McDougle L, et al. Implicit racial bias in medical school admissions. Acad Med 2017;92(3):365–9.

41. Clark M, Rothstein J, Schanzenbach DW. Selection bias in college admissions test scores. Econ Educ Rev 2009;28(3):295–307.

42. Polanco-Santana JC, Storino A, Souza-Mota L, et al. Ethnic/racial bias in medical school performance evaluation of general surgery residency applicants. J Surg Educ 2021-Oct;78(5):1524–34.

43. Ceppa DP, Antonoff MA, Tong BC, et al. Women in thoracic surgery update on the status of women in cardiothoracic surgery. Ann Thorac Surg 2022; 113(3):918–25.

44. Pompili C, Opitz I, Backhus L, et al. The impact of gender bias in cardiothoracic surgery in Europe: European Society of Thoracic Surgeons and European Association for Cardio-Thoracic Surgery survey. Eur J Cardio Thorac Surg 2022;61(6):1390–9.

45. Peck CJ, Roberts SE, Ly CL, et al. Embracing allyship in academic surgery: How all surgeons can become effective champions for change. JACS 2022;235:371–4.

46. Wood DE. How can men be good allies for women in surgery? #HeForShe. J Thorac Dis 2021;13(1): 492–501.

47. Martinez S, Araj J, Reid S, et al. Allyship in Residency: An introductory module on medical allyship for graduate medical trainees. MedEdPORTAL 2021;17:11200.

48. Weaver JL, Cannada L, Anand T, et al, Association of Women Surgeons Publications Committee. The importance of allyship in academic surgery. Am J Surg 2023;225(4):805–7.

49. Donington JS, Litle VR, Sesti J, et al. The WTS report on the current status of women in cardiothoracic surgery. Ann Thorac Surg 2012;94(2):452–8 [discussion 458-9].

50. Trudell A, Frankel W, Luc J, et al. Enhancing support for women in cardiothoracic surgery through allyship and targeted initiatives. Ann Thorac Surg 2022;113: 1676–84.

51. Rodriguez J, Campbell K, Poloi L. Addressing disparities in academic medicine: What of the minority tax? BMC Med Educ 2015;15:6.

52. Edwards MA. Diversity in the cardiothoracic surgery workforce: What can I do. Thorac Surg Clin 2024; 34(1):89–97.

53. Cooke DT, Olive J, Godoy L, et al. The importance of a diverse specialty: Introducing the STS Workforce on Diversity and Inclusion. Ann Thorac Surg 2019; 108(4):1000–5.

54. Corsini EM, Olive JK, Antonoff MM. The current status and importance of diversity in cardiothoracic surgery. Current Surgery Reports 2020;8(9).

55. Perdomo D, Pebworth R, Lawton JS, et al. The society of thoracic surgeons looking to the future scholarship program: a 15-year review. Ann Thorac Surg 2023;21. S0003-S4975(23)00966-9.

56. Khalil S, Olds A, Chin K, et al. Implementation of well-being for cardiothoracic surgeons. Thorac Surg Clin 2024;34(1):63–76.

57. Eisenberg MA, Deboever N, Swisher SG, et al. Removing implicit bias from cardiothoracic surgery resident recruitment: Changing the paradigm. J Surg Res 2023;292:72–8.

History and Current Status of Well-being Among Organizations (Impact of Wellness on a Section, Division, Institution and Profession, ACGME Requirements, Policies)

Anna Olds, MD[a,*], Anastasiia Tompkins, BS, BA[b], Cherie P. Erkmen, MD[c]

KEYWORDS

• Well-being • Burnout • Diversity • Inclusion • Policy

KEY POINTS

- Burnout is prevalent among cardiothoracic surgeons and trainees.
- The American Association for Thoracic Surgery, The Society of Thoracic Surgeons, Women in Thoracic Surgery, Thoracic Surgery Directors Association, and Thoracic Surgery Resident Associationhave all developed initiatives to combat burnout, but more work is needed.
- Professional organizations and institutions should improve access to wellness resources and implement policies to encourage wellness and prevent burnout among trainees and surgeons.
- Encouraging inclusion of surgeons with underrepresented genders, races, ethnicities, religions, and sexual orientations is vital to promoting the culture of wellness.
- There are small attainable changes that programs and departments can make that will have noticeable improvements in trainee and surgeon well-being.

INTRODUCTION

Since burnout was described in the 1970s, significant progress has been made in studying the contributing factors and consequences of burnout in the medical field. Those in surgical specialties, particularly cardiothoracic surgery, may be at higher risk of burnout because of the associated requirements and difficulties of the profession. Burnout adversely impacts individual surgeon, their patients, their institutions, and the cardiothoracic community as a whole. Strides to address burnout and improve physician well-being have been taken by the American Medical Association and the Accreditation Council for Graduate Medical Education (ACGME) to advance access to wellness resources for physicians both in training and in practice. Cardiothoracic surgical organizations have developed wellness committees and task forces to provide resources, open discussions, and study burnout within the specialty. Additionally, the American Board of Thoracic Surgery (ABTS) along with the Thoracic Surgery Directors Association (TSDA) and the Thoracic Surgery

[a] Department of Surgery, University of Southern California, 1520 San Pablo Street, Suite 4300, Los Angeles, CA 90033, USA; [b] Center for Asian Health, Lewis Katz School of Medicine at Temple University, 3401 N. Broad Street, Suite 501, Philadelphia, PA, USA; [c] Department of Thoracic Medicine and Surgery, Temple University Hospital, 3401 N. Broad Street, Suite 501, Philadelphia, PA 19140, USA
* Corresponding author. 1520 San Pablo Street, Suite 4300, Los Angeles, CA 90033.
E-mail address: anna.olds@med.usc.edu

Thorac Surg Clin 34 (2024) 249–259
https://doi.org/10.1016/j.thorsurg.2024.04.003
1547-4127/24/© 2024 Elsevier Inc. All rights reserved.

Resident Association (TSRA) has developed policies and resources focused on cardiothoracic surgery trainees to improve well-being and protect against burnout. However, significant work is still needed, as a recent survey in 2022 demonstrated significant burnout, depression, and a lack of wellness resources for many surgeons around the country. This article provides an overview of data surrounding well-being and burnout in cardiothoracic surgery, policies and interventions that have been initiated to combat burnout, and responses to interventions.

HISTORY OF BURNOUT IN THE MEDICAL FIELD

Burnout was initially described and investigated in the 1970s in relation to psychologists and their emotional fatigue around their work but is now studied across many different jobs and settings.[1,2] Burnout can be measured using multiple scales, with the most popular being the Maslach Burnout Inventory, which measures emotional exhaustion, depersonalization, and other relevant factors.[2–4] In the healthcare realm, research has recently increased surrounding burnout in the setting of the coronavirus disease 2019 (COVID-19) pandemic. Even before COVID-19, researchers were referring to burnout in the healthcare professions a "crisis" with multiple calls to action, especially because of high rates of physician suicide.[1,5] The prevalence of burnout among United States (US) physicians has been quoted around 35% to 55% in most studies, with some as high as 80%, and has been shown to have negative impacts on patient care errors, outcomes, healthcare costs, and physician health.[3,6–11] Physician burnout has consistently been shown to be higher than the general working US population.[7,12] One survey of US physicians and the general working population published in 2022 found that physicians are at approximately 40% increased risk of burnout and approximately 30% less likely to be satisfied with work life balance than the general working population.[7]

A systematic review published in 2022 examining burnout predictors found that job autonomy and control, support from leadership, better work-life balance, and having a spouse along with personal social support are all associated with less burnout.[1] (**Fig. 1**) These factors have been noted in multiple other studies as well.[3,9] (see **Fig. 1**) One recent review acknowledges 6 primary principles of well-being: progress toward a goal, actions aligned with mission, connectedness, social relatedness, safety, and autonomy.[13] (see **Fig. 1**) Primary care specialties and certain

surgical subspecialties have been noted to have the highest rates of burnout, and women physicians appear to be at a higher risk for burnout than their male colleagues.[1,7–9,14] These same findings have been demonstrated in residents, who often have higher rates of burnout than attendings.[9,12] Within general surgical training, Hu and colleagues published results from a survey of surgical residents after the American Board of Surgery in-training examination (ABSITE) in 2018, which demonstrated that 38.5% of surgical residents felt burnout weekly at minimum and 4.5% had suicidal thoughts in the year before.[15] Furthermore, Yue-Yung and colleagues published a striking manuscript from this same survey in 2018 detailing the high prevalence of abuse of surgical residents by both patients and their attendings.[15] Despite increased levels of burnout, however, physicians have been shown to display higher resilience than the general US working population, which can be protective against burnout.[16]

Implementing work hour restrictions for residents was a pivotal step in the direction of improved wellness for physicians. A shift in physician training paradigms led to a series of interventions to address the epidemic of physician burnout and suicide. Mandated resident work hour restrictions started in New York State in the 1990s after the case of Libby Zion, and they were made official by the Accreditation Council for Graduate Medical Education (ACGME) for all US residency programs in 2003. These restrictions included one period of 24 hours off duty per week averaged over 4 weeks, no more than once every 3 nights of call, and a limit of 80 hours per week including education time.[17] In 2010, after research demonstrated that significant fatigue occurs with over 30 hours of time awake, the ACGME further restricted work hours. These new restrictions started in 2011, which included a 16-h duty limit for interns and a required 14 hours off duty after a 24-h call period for senior residents.[17] After the resident work hour restrictions were introduced, a significant amount of controversy arose regarding whether residents would complete residency as well-trained as those without hour restrictions. Concern about preparedness for practice can impact well-being of both faculty and trainees. Hour restrictions have been maintained, but policymakers realized that more than just sleep deprivation factors into burnout and wellness at the training level and at the attending physician level.

BURNOUT IN CARDIOTHORACIC SURGERY

Although there has been a significant amount of effort to combat burnout in medicine over the

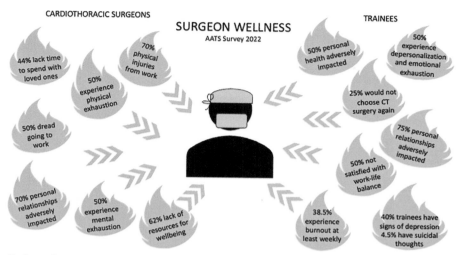

Fig. 1. Cardiothoracic surgeon experience regarding wellness and burnout, including attending surgeons and trainees.

past several decades, the surgical subspecialties have recently become more interested in studying burnout. Surgeons may experience increased levels of burnout compared with other specialties because of a variety of factors, which is associated with increased surgical errors and decreased job satisfaction.[9,18] The data are not as robust for cardiothoracic surgery as for other surgical specialties. A well-being survey for cardiothoracic surgeons was designed and distributed in 2021 by the American Association for Thoracic Surgery (AATS) Wellness Committee.[19] Not surprisingly, approximately 50% of respondents dreaded going to work, experienced physical and mental exhaustion at work, and lacked enthusiasm at work. Additionally, 44% of surgeons felt that they lacked enough time to spend with loved ones, which affected women more than men (**Fig. 2**). Younger surgeons with children less than 19 year old were more likely to report burnout, and 70% of surgeons reported that their personal relationships were impacted by burnout. Neck or back problems attributed to a surgical career affected 70% of surgeons, with women suffering more injuries. Unfortunately, 62% of respondents had a lack of wellness and supportive resources at their workplaces, while those who had access to these resources experienced significantly less burnout. These numbers are similar to burnout rates in other medical specialties, demonstrating opportunities for improvement.[3,6–11]

Studies examining burnout and wellness among cardiothoracic surgery trainees have found similar results. Chow and colleagues surveyed all US cardiothoracic trainees, finding that greater than 50% of trainees were not satisfied with their

personal and work life balance and greater than 25% would not choose cardiothoracic surgery again.[20] (see **Fig. 2**) Over 40% had signs of depression and greater than 50% had signs of emotional exhaustion and depersonalization, which are criteria for burnout.[20] Furthermore, training negatively impacted personal health for greater than 50% of trainees, and personal relationships for greater than 75% of trainees.[20] Female trainees and those with children were more likely to regret choosing cardiothoracic surgery as a specialty. Cardiothoracic surgical trainees are at extremely high risk of burnout because of the arduous nature of the specialty. Long hours, difficult and exhausting call schedules, frequent overnight emergencies, and long duration of training put cardiothoracic surgery trainees at higher risk of burnout than other specialties.[21] Additionally, the culture of cardiothoracic surgical training values personal responsibility, which can lead to feelings of isolation.[21] After training, at the beginning of independent practice, there are several significant contributors to burnout including lack of knowledge about the financial aspects of medicine, as well as lack of education and resources to combat burnout in practice.[22,23]

Cardiothoracic surgery tends to attract highly motivated, driven people, but this can come at the price of exclusivity. Perceptions of exclusion, whether resulting from outright bias or unconscious biases, can lead to and perpetuate burnout, negativity, self-doubt, and feelings of isolation.[24–26] Exclusivity leads to lack of interconnectedness with others and a lack of safety, clashing with the principles of well-being.[13] Perceptions of exclusivity are noted in relation to underrepresentation or differences in gender, sexual orientation, race or

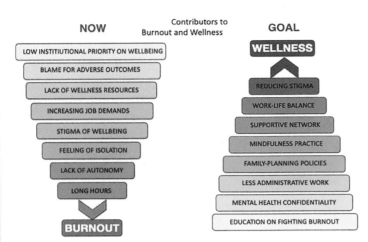

Fig. 2. Factors contributing to wellness and burnout, providing areas for potential intervention.

ethnicity, religion, etc.[24,25,27] Women and racial and ethnic minorities remain underrepresented in cardiothoracic surgery, especially in academia, and discrimination because of gender or race has been found in 83% of Black and 39% of Asian surgeons versus 27% of White surgeons.[24,28–30] Several reports have found that several women cardiothoracic surgeons (some studies reporting approximately 75%) believe that cardiothoracic surgery is not a welcoming environment for women, while a low proportion of men surgeons perceive this (approximately 25%).[25,31–33] In 2019, the Society of Thoracic Surgeons (STS) Ad Hoc Presidential Task Force on Diversity and Inclusion published results from a survey of STS members designed to study perceptions and perspectives of diversity and inclusion in cardiothoracic surgery.[34] They found that 24% of respondents believed the myth that diversity is a pipeline problem, and 18% believed that diversity does not support merit, while 15% of respondents believed that disparities are not present in the field and that there is nothing to address.[34] This highlights the need for more strategies to promote awareness of biases, acknowledge the value of diversity, and create a culture of inclusion for all cardiothoracic surgeons and trainees.

CURRENT EFFORTS TO COMBAT BURNOUT
Broad Efforts Within Medicine

To combat burnout in US physicians, there have been efforts to create educational and supportive resources by many organizations, associations, and foundations (**Table 1**). In particular, the American Medical Association (AMA) has developed several interventions and policies.[35,36] Importantly, the AMA advocates for legislation that supports and increases physician wellness resource

accessibility and confidentiality for physicians who use them. The AMA successfully campaigned for the Dr Lorna Breen Health Care Provider Protection Act to be signed into law in 2022. This legislation provides grant money to train medical professionals in strategies to reduce and prevent burnout and includes a national campaign that focuses on encouragement for struggling physicians to seek help. With the help of the AMA, laws in Virginia, Arizona, Indiana, and South Dakota have been passed to protect physician and medical student confidentiality in receiving care for burnout and wellness. At the individual physician level, the AMA has many online resources on its website, as well as its STEPS Forward toolkits for wellness.[35,36] In an initiative geared toward organizations and health systems, the AMA developed the Joy in Medicine Health System Recognition Program, which helps organizations improve healthcare practitioner wellness and decrease burnout. Lastly, the AMA sponsors 2 large conferences focused on physician well-being and burnout, entitled the International Conference on Physician Health and the American Conference on Physician Health.[35,36]

There have been significant strides to protect and advocate for trainee wellness in the past several decades. The ACGME, Association of American Medical Colleges, and National Academy of Medicine developed a "Clinician Well-Being and Resilience" program in 2017 to increase education on physician burnout, improve organizational methods to combat burnout, and evaluate efficacy of interventions.[21] Over 200 institutions joined this collaborative and have participated in efforts to improve physician well-being.[37] The ACGME strongly advocates for protection of vacation and leave time for residents to foster work-life

Table 1
Available resources

Resource	Link
AMA STEPs Forward Toolkits	https://edhub.ama-assn.org/steps-forward/pages/professional-well-being
The Dr. Lorna Breen Heroes Foundation	https://drlornabreen.org
Joy in Medicine Health System Recognition Program	https://www.ama-assn.org/practice-management/physician-health/ama-joy-medicine-health-system-recognition-program
the International Conference on Physician Health	https://www.ama-assn.org/about/events/international-conference-physician-health
the American Conference on Physician Health	https://www.physician-well-being-conference.org
Clinician Well-Being and Resilience" program	https://nam.edu/initiatives/clinician-resilience-and-well-being/
ACGME AWARE Well-Being Resources	https://dl.acgme.org/pages/well-being
Mindfulness-based interventions	Waking Up app, Calm app, Insight Timer app
AATS Wellness Committee	https://www.aats.org/the-wellness-corner
STS Workforce on Wellness	https://www.sts.org/resources/life-career/wellness-resources
STS Aspiring CT Surgeons Blog - A Space for Trainees	https://www.sts.org/publications/aspiring-ct-surgeons-blog-space-trainees
STS Career Development Blog	https://www.sts.org/topics/career-development-blog
"The Resilient Surgeon" Podcast	https://www.sts.org/topics/resilient-surgeon
The Women in Thoracic Surgery (mentoring programs, scholarships)	https://wtsnet.org
TSRA & TSDA Wellness Webinar Series	https://soundcloud.com/tsrapodcast/tsratsda-wellness-webinar-dealing-with-complications

balance.[38] Current ACGME policy dictates that all residency programs must provide 6 weeks minimum of paid leave for parental, caregiver, or medical leave.[38] The ACGME Program Requirements include a section on Well-Being that requires programs to be accountable for "scheduling, work intensity, and work compression that impacts residents' well-being" and to prioritize the safety of residents and attendings.[38] Additionally, programs are required to put into place "policies and programs that encourage optimal resident and faculty member well-being" including time away from work for social connection, physical activity, medical appointments, and self-care. ACGME policies also require education about the symptoms and signs of burnout and access to resources for self-care, burnout screening, and treatment. Additionally, the ACGME website provides well-being resources for programs, including articles, lectures, and guidebooks for generating well-being focused programs.[38]

Various publications have investigated the impact of specific interventions to combat burnout and improve wellness (see **Fig. 2**). Mindfulness-based interventions, especially those that are both accessible and impactful for physicians, have demonstrated significant positive impacts on physician wellness in several systematic reviews and trials wellness.[39–43] Mindfulness is an awareness of the present, focusing on the breath, and attempting to be present without judgment, and includes mindfulness-based stress reduction (MBSR) techniques.[39,40,44] Mindfulness-based interventions can significantly decrease burnout scores, reduce stress, and improve overall well-being.[39–41,45] Interventions directed by the organization may have significantly more improvement compared with individually directed interventions to combat burnout, suggesting that this requires organization level intervention.[42] Work hour limits, self-care workshops, and mindfulness-based interventions have all been shown to decrease burnout in residents specifically.[46,47]

Efforts Specific to Cardiothoracic Surgery

Multiple surgeon wellness initiatives have also been started within cardiothoracic surgery. At annual AATS and STS meetings, there are an increasing number of well-being sessions to foster discussion about potential interventions and improvements. The AATS recently developed a Wellness Committee whose focus is to "improve the physical and mental well-being of members by developing wellness sessions for the Annual Meeting, providing wellness-related content for the AATS Newsletter, and handling issues surrounding the culture of safety and/or decorum."[48] In addition to completing and publishing a wellness and burnout survey of cardiothoracic surgeons, the committee has also hosted webinars focused on well-being. These include webinars to provide education to young surgeons and trainees about topics such as the details of an academic career to help trainees make career decisions according to their personal and professional goals. The STS has also developed a Workforce on Wellness.[49] The STS Workforce on Diversity, Equity, and Inclusion (DEI) has also done a significant amount of work on studying and combatting burnout.[50] The DEI Workforce advocates for inclusion of all genders, races, ethnicities, religions, and sexual orientations at the trainee level, attending surgeon level, and within the academic hierarchy. Over the last several years, these committees have published numerous manuscripts, blog posts, and articles on wellness topics. The STS has several blogs, including the Aspiring CT Surgeons blog for medical students and trainees, a Career Development Blog for trainees and early career surgeons, and clinical blogs for residents and attending surgeons. Examples of blog topics include personal finance, ergonomics for surgeons, and fertility in cardiothoracic surgery, dealing with complications, overcoming career setbacks, and numerous posts during the COVID-19 pandemic to coach surgeons through difficult times.

The STS also sponsors "The Resilient Surgeon" podcast, which was developed by Dr Michael Maddaus, a thoracic surgeon and a member of the STS Workforce on Wellness. Dr Maddaus records episodes with high-achieving people inside and outside of cardiothoracic surgery to provide resources, educate about strategies to combat burnout, or feature someone who shares personal experience on burnout. As of August 2023, there were 154 podcasts, which are freely available for surgeons and trainees through the STS website.[49] Dr Maddaus also hosts the Resilient Surgeon newsletter subscription to "inspire surgeons to be their best selves and lead fulfilling lives, in and out of the operating room."[49] The newsletter provides guidance through discussion of topics like meta-awareness, mindfulness, and interpersonal skills.[49] The WTS organization has also increased its focus on wellness and burnout among women surgeons.

The organization provides mentoring programs for women trainees and early career surgeons and offers a network of women who are focused on helping each other succeed. There have been many initiatives led by the WTS focused on gender equality, diversity, and wellness, including publications detailing strategies to improve the support of women trainees and practicing surgeons.[31–33,51] Additionally, the WTS scholarship programs assist women and minority groups in attending national meetings and match them with WTS mentors. These scholarship programs have been shown to improve career trajectories and productivity.[52]

In addition to AATS, STS, and WTS efforts to improve well-being, there have been several policy updates specifically for trainees in cardiothoracic surgery. As research has shown, younger surgeons, specifically women, with children are at highest risk for burnout. Furthermore, it is well-documented that women surgeons experience significantly higher rates of pregnancy complication and infertility than the general population.[53–57] Accordingly, there have been improvements in parental, medical, and caregiver leave policies in recent years. In 2020, the ABTS updated the leave policies for cardiothoracic surgery trainees to offer better work-life balance, family building, and personal time during long and arduous training.[58] Trainees in traditional or '4 + 3' pathways can take a single 6-week period of time for leave in addition to vacation time. Integrated trainees may take 2 6-week periods off for leave. Congenital subspecialty fellows may take 6 weeks.[58]

A 2019 survey by the TSDA demonstrated that many cardiothoracic surgery program directors are unaware of available trainee wellness resources.[22] The TSDA is invested in increasing resources and accessibility to wellness resources for trainees. A joint AATS and TSDA committee focuses on developing institutional guidelines for trainee wellness and promoting research on wellness.[22] The STS DEI Workforce also partnered with TSDA to send welcome letters to new cardiothoracic surgery trainees, which included wellness resources. This workforce has sponsored a podcast series entitled "Same Surgeon, Different Light" featuring surgeons from different backgrounds to discuss their stories, personal struggles, and diverse backgrounds. TSRA has also been involved in numerous national surveys and publications detailing the status of well-being among trainees and highlighting aspects of training that need to change to improve wellness.

TSRA and TSDA are working to improve access to wellness resources for training programs, program directors, faculty, and trainees. Dedicated to opening discussions about well-being and burnout, TSRA and TSDA created a Wellness Webinar Series in 2023. These webinars are available to everyone in the cardiothoracic surgery community, but focus specifically on well-being issues impacting trainees, students, and early career surgeons. Topics include dealing with complications, personal finance, starting a family in training or as a young attending, among others. The webinars are broadcasted live with panels that include trainees and senior surgeons, as well as financial advisors and others outside of medicine who have insight that could help trainees navigate these issues. All webinars are recorded and posted into an online bank where they are accessible to residency programs and trainees. The webinar bank can be found on the TSRA YouTube page or WebApp (see **Table 1**).

ASPIRATIONAL EFFORTS TO COMBAT BURNOUT AND IMPROVE WELLNESS

In the general medical community, the AMA is working to decrease stigma associated with seeking help for burnout. The organization advocates for laws supporting confidentiality for medical students and physicians seeking mental health treatment. This involves urging state licensing boards, health systems, and credentialing boards to maintain physician confidentiality regarding treatment, and remove questions relating to mental health, substance use, etc.[35,36] The goal is to have credentialing, licensing, and employing committees only ask questions pertaining to current mental health and ability to practice, and to not ask probing questions about past mental health treatment, as this may deter physicians from seeking help. The AMA is also advocating for reduction in administrative tasks, which are shown in numerous studies to increase burnout.[35,36] Additionally, there is advocacy for physician wellness reporting systems and programs for physicians to seek help.

Within the general surgical community, an active clinical trial for residency programs entitled the Surgical Education Culture Optimization through targeted interventions based on National comparative Data trial began enrolling and collecting data in 2019.[15,20,59] This trial has enrolled over 200 programs and randomized them to the control arm, which generates an annual report on their residents' burnout and well-being data compared with other US programs versus intervention arm, which generates a detailed report of resident well-being with access to Wellness Toolkits.[59] The results of this trial may help inform residency programs about tools and strategies for improving resident wellness and burnout.

In 2023, the Association of Women Surgeons (AWS) published a "Comprehensive Initiative for Healthy Surgical Families During Residency and Fellowship Training" that can serve as a guide for cardiothoracic surgery programs.[60] The AWS guide suggests the following: trainees should plan ahead, if possible, for parenthood, program directors should support family planning and create a culture of inclusivity and support, and programs should provide information and access to infertility and reproductive treatments, as well as mental health resources.[60] It is imperative to provide protections for residents wishing to start families, including both childbearing and non-childbearing residents who are parents. Institutional support will help to lessen burnout in the long run. Although some institutions provide financial support and encouragement for woman trainees and attendees to participate in egg harvesting or in vitro fertilization, this is rare and is an area for improvement. Additionally, many institutions do not have affordable childcare for trainees or early career surgeons, increasing the potential for financial strain and burnout.[19,60] Affordable accessible childcare is also recommended by Bremner and colleagues in the AATS Wellness Committee survey to lessen burnout.[19]

Several institutions have developed more specific wellness-focused parental leave policies for their cardiothoracic surgery training programs. Possibly the most progressive example of this is from the University of Michigan.[56] The University of Michigan's leadership recently published their evidence-based policies around childbearing residents, with a focus on protecting the health of the pregnant resident while also fostering a culture of teamwork and shared responsibility.[56] Prenatally, trainees are excused for all medical appointments. In the case of pregnancy complications or hyperemesis gravidarum, the policy specifies that "if the trainee experiences severe cramping or bleeding at any time while on duty, arrangements will be made to facilitate transport for care" with scheduling adjustments being the responsibility of the chief resident or program director, not the pregnant trainee. Pregnant trainees in their third trimester are limited to working less than or equal to 12 consecutive hours, and no overnight calls.[56] Postnatally, both men and women trainees are encouraged to take parental leave. They have implemented a pre-planned system for coverage of critical portions of cases to allow breastfeeding residents to leave clinical duties to pump without interruptions to patient care.[56] This system depends on teamwork and support from other residents, advanced practitioners, and faculty. Importantly, these University of Michigan policies have

Box 1	
Action items for professional societies	

Advocate for legislation protecting physicians from mandatory mental health treatment reporting for licensing.

Implement industry standard that no medical or psychiatric history is required for licensing unless it pertains to current function.

Require formalized burnout screening for training programs, and train program directors in screening mechanisms.

Require mindfulness-based intervention accessibility for training programs.

Continue to research burnout, improve access to resources, and advocate for change on the institutional and organizational level.

Participate in AMA initiatives to improve access to burnout resources and encourage struggling surgeons to seek help.

Develop an accessible peer support program for surgeons struggling with burnout.

Offer mindfulness-based interventions and resilience training as workshops or programs for surgeons through STS/AATS.

Develop physical therapy/ergonomics workshops and resources to improve musculoskeletal health, normalize seeking help for musculoskeletal pain.

Require formalized policies from training programs to protect trainees starting families.

Continue to make wellness a key portion of annual meetings.

Abbreviations: AMA, American Medical Association; MSK, musculoskeletal; PT, physical therapy.

Box 2	
Action items at the institutional and departmental levels	

Improve, maintain, and confirm access to confidential mental health resources for trainees and attending surgeons.

Nominate a wellness officer within the institution with responsibilities to educate and screen for burnout, and improve resources for employees.

Provide accessible and affordable childcare options for trainees and attendings, as surgeons with young children are at highest risk of burnout.

Develop and implement organized, specific policies to protect trainees starting families.

Provide education and affordable access to family planning and fertility resources for trainees and attending surgeons.

Provide affordable well-being resources (courses, workshops, emotional support, psychotherapy, exercise courses, mindfulness meditation groups, and retreats) to trainees and attendings.

Mandate that each trainee and attending receive a detailed list of all mental/physical health resources available and how to find them.

Provide accessible professional coaching and MBSR training for attending surgeons whether through individual institutions or through AATS/STS.

Improve education during training on transitioning from trainee to attending to better prepare early career surgeons for inevitable challenges.

Provide access to physical therapy and places to exercise to encourage physical fitness and encourage trainees and surgeons to seek help for musculoskeletal pain.

Offer affordable and healthy food options for trainees and attending surgeons to maintain physical well-being.

Abbreviation: MBSR, mindfulness based stress reduction.

not impacted or worsened quality of training, as this is often cited as a reason to avoid such policies.[56] The University of Michigan policies can serve as an example of what is possible in cardiothoracic surgery training to foster work-life integration and support residents in starting families.

Mindfulness-based interventions, like formal mindfulness-based stress reduction training, and professional coaching are current areas of study in cardiothoracic surgeons.[39,45,61] Data on professional resilience coaching show statistically significant improvement in resilience, measured on a validated Brief Resilience Scale.[61] This could be accomplished on a small scale as a workshop or short program and could be implemented in training programs. To combat burnout, Bremner and colleagues recommend that institutions

provide emotional support resources to surgeons in the form of peer support programs and coaching programs.[19] Mindfulness training may be valuable for decreasing burnout, and providing access to physical therapy to mitigate the physical injuries associated with surgery may help lessen burnout. Recently, the focus of wellness interventions has shifted from the individual to institutions and professional societies. Institutional and organizational strategies are likely to have the most impact in surgeon wellness. Actions including making burnout assessment tools available and developing policies for intervention and treatment of burnout require institutional investment in the well-being of physicians.[22] Residency programs, cardiothoracic surgery leadership, and organizations should aim for evidence-based changes that are relevant to their trainees and faculty (**Boxes 1** and **2**).

CLINICS ARE POINTS

- Wellness is important for patient care, efficiency, and recruitment of the best and brightest to the field of cardiothoracic surgery.
- Wellness initiatives in medicine overall have improved in the past several decades, but more work is needed in cardiothoracic surgery.
- The cardiothoracic surgery organizations have improved efforts to combat burnout but bigger and more concrete initiatives are needed.
- Burnout is prevalent in cardiothoracic surgeons and trainees and is related to lack of inclusion, inability to balance personal life, and lack of autonomy, among other factors.
- Policies and efforts at the individual level are important, but institutional and organizational efforts are necessary and may be more impactful.

DISCLOSURE

The authors have nothing to disclose.

REFERENCES

1. Meredith LS, Bouskill K, Chang J, et al. Predictors of burnout among US healthcare providers: a systematic review. BMJ Open 2022;12(8). https://doi.org/10.1136/bmjopen-2021-054243.
2. Maslach C, Schaufeli WB and Leiter MP. JOB BURNOUT, Available at: www.annualreviews.org, (Accessed November 8, 2023), 2000.
3. West CP, Dyrbye LN, Shanafelt TD. Physician burnout: contributors, consequences and solutions. J Intern Med 2018;283(6):516–29.
4. Maslach CSEJ and MPLeiter. Maslach burnout Inventory. 3rd edition. Consulting Psychologists Press; 1996.
5. Dzau VJ, Kirch DG, Nasca TJ. To Care Is Human — Collectively Confronting the Clinician-Burnout Crisis. N Engl J Med 2018;378(4):312–4.
6. Han S, Shanafelt TD, Sinsky CA, et al. Estimating the attributable cost of physician burnout in the United States. Ann Intern Med 2019;170(11):784–90.
7. Shanafelt TD, West CP, Sinsky C, et al. Changes in Burnout and Satisfaction With Work-Life Integration in Physicians and the General US Working Population Between 2011 and 2020. Mayo Clin Proc 2022;97(3):491–506.
8. West CP, Dyrbye LN, Erwin PJ, et al. Interventions to prevent and reduce physician burnout: a systematic review and meta-analysis. Lancet 2016;388(10057):2272–81.
9. Dyrbye LN, Burke SE, Hardeman RR, et al. Association of clinical specialty with symptoms of burnout and career choice regret among US resident physicians. JAMA, J Am Med Assoc 2018;320(11):1114–30.
10. Rotenstein LS, Torre M, Ramos MA, et al. Prevalence of burnout among physicians a systematic review. JAMA, J Am Med Assoc 2018;320(11):1131–50.
11. Rothenberger DA. Physician Burnout and Well-Being: A Systematic Review and Framework for Action. Dis Colon Rectum 2017;60(6):567–76.
12. Dyrbye LN, West CP, Satele D, et al. Burnout among u.s. medical students, residents, and early career physicians relative to the general u.s. population. Acad Med 2014;89(3):443–51.
13. Khalil S, Olds A, Chin K, et al. Implementation of Well-Being for Cardiothoracic Surgeons. Thorac Surg Clin 2024;34(1):63–76.
14. Linzer M, Jin JO, Shah P, et al. Trends in Clinician Burnout with Associated Mitigating and Aggravating Factors during the COVID-19 Pandemic. JAMA Health Forum 2022;3(11):E224163.
15. Hu YY, Ellis RJ, Hewitt DB, et al. Discrimination, Abuse, Harassment, and Burnout in Surgical Residency Training. N Engl J Med 2019;381(18):1741–52.
16. West CP, Dyrbye LN, Sinsky C, et al. Resilience and Burnout among Physicians and the General US Working Population. JAMA Netw Open 2020;3(7). https://doi.org/10.1001/jamanetworkopen.2020.9385.
17. Fabricant PD, Dy CJ, Dare DM, et al. A Narrative Review of Surgical Resident Duty Hour Limits: Where Do We Go From Here? J Grad Med Educ 2013;5(1):19–24.
18. Shanafelt TD, Balch CM, Bechamps G, et al. Burnout and medical errors among American surgeons. Ann Surg 2010;251(6):995–1000.
19. Bremner RM, Ungerleider RM, Ungerleider J, et al. Well-being of Cardiothoracic Surgeons in the Time of COVID-19: A Survey by the Wellness Committee of the American Association for Thoracic Surgery. Semin Thorac Cardiovasc Surg 2022. https://doi.org/10.1053/j.semtcvs.2022.10.002.

20. Chow OS, Sudarshan M, Maxfield MW, et al. National Survey of Burnout and Distress Among Cardiothoracic Surgery Trainees. Ann Thorac Surg 2021;111:2066–71.

21. Swain JBD, Soegaard Ballester JM, Luc JGY, et al. Burning the candle at both ends: Mitigating surgeon burnout at the training stages. J Thorac Cardiovasc Surg 2021;162(2):637–42.

22. Fajardo R, Vaporciyan A, Starnes S, et al. Cardiothoracic surgery wellness: Now and the formidable road ahead. J Thorac Cardiovasc Surg 2021; 161(1):333–7.

23. Fiedler AG, Sihag S. Entering the great unknown: Transition to academic practice. J Thorac Cardiovasc Surg 2020;159(3):1156–60.

24. Erhunmwunsee L, Backhus LM, Godoy L, et al. Report from the Workforce on Diversity and Inclusion—The Society of Thoracic Surgeons Members' Bias Experiences. Ann Thorac Surg 2019;108(5): 1287–91.

25. Backhus LM, Lui NS, Cooke DT, et al. Unconscious Bias: Addressing the Hidden Impact on Surgical Education. Thorac Surg Clin 2019;29(3):259–67.

26. Erkmen CP, Ortmeyer KA, Pelletier GJ, et al. An Approach to Diversity and Inclusion in Cardiothoracic Surgery. Ann Thorac Surg 2021;111(3): 747–52.

27. Backhus LM, Fann BE, Hui DS, et al. Culture of Safety and Gender Inclusion in Cardiothoracic Surgery. Ann Thorac Surg 2018;106(4):951–8.

28. Ceppa DKP. Social Disparities in the Thoracic Surgery Workforce. Thorac Surg Clin 2022;32(1):103–9.

29. Godoy LA, Hill E, Cooke DT. Social Disparities in Thoracic Surgery Education. Thorac Surg Clin 2022;32(1):91–102.

30. Ortmeyer KA, Raman V, Tiko-Okoye C, et al. Women and Minorities Underrepresented in Academic Cardiothoracic Surgery: It's Time for Next Steps. Ann Thorac Surg 2021;112(4):1349–55.

31. Giuliano K, Ceppa DKP, Antonoff M, et al. Women in Thoracic Surgery 2020 Update—Subspecialty and Work-Life Balance Analysis. Ann Thorac Surg 2022;114:1933–42.

32. Ceppa DKP, Antonoff MB, Tong BC, et al. 2020 Women in Thoracic Surgery Update on the Status of Women in Cardiothoracic Surgery. Ann Thorac Surg 2022;113:918–25.

33. Preventza O, Backhus L. US women in thoracic surgery: Reflections on the past and opportunities for the future. J Thorac Dis 2021;13(1):473–9.

34. Backhus LM, Kpodonu J, Romano JC, et al. An Exploration of Myths, Barriers, and Strategies for Improving Diversity Among STS Members. Ann Thorac Surg 2019;108(6):1617–24.

35. American Medical Association. AMA physician well-being program. AMA website. 2023. Available at: www.ama-assn.org.

36. American Medical Association. AMA fights causes of physician burnout. AMA website. 2023. Available at: www.ama-assn.org.

37. NAM change maker campaign for health workforce well-being. National Academy of Medicine website. 2023. Available at: https://nam.edu/initiatives/clinician-resilience-and-well-being/change-makers/.

38. ACGME Common Program Requirements (Residency). Accreditation Council for Graduate Medical Education website; 2023. www.acgme.org/OsteopathicRecognition.

39. Fendel JC, Bürkle JJ, Göritz AS. Mindfulness-based interventions to reduce burnout and stress in physicians: A study protocol for a systematic review and meta-analysis. BMJ Open 2019;9(11). https://doi.org/10.1136/bmjopen-2019-032295.

40. Fendel JC, Bürkle JJ, Göritz AS. Mindfulness-Based Interventions to Reduce Burnout and Stress in Physicians: A Systematic Review and Meta-Analysis. Acad Med 2021;96(5):751–64.

41. Goodman MJ, Schorling JB. A mindfulness course decreases burnout and improves well-being among healthcare providers. Int J Psychiatry Med 2012; 43(2):119–28.

42. Panagioti M, Panagopoulou E, Bower P, et al. Controlled interventions to reduce burnout in physicians a systematic review and meta-analysis. JAMA Intern Med 2017;177(2):195–205.

43. Naviaux AF, Barbier L, Chopinet S, et al. Ways of preventing surgeon burnout. J Visc Surg 2023;160(1):33–8.

44. Kabat-Zinn J. Coming to Our Senses: Healing Ourselves and the World through mindfulness. Hachette Books; 2005.

45. Maddaus M. The Resilience Bank Account: Skills for Optimal Performance. Ann Thorac Surg 2020; 109(1):18–25.

46. Busireddy KR, Miller JA, Ellison K, et al. Efficacy of Interventions to Reduce Resident Physician Burnout: A Systematic Review. J Grad Med Educ 2017;9(3): 294–301.

47. Lebares CC, Coaston TN, Delucchi KL, et al. Enhanced Stress Resilience Training in Surgeons: Iterative Adaptation and Biopsychosocial Effects in 2 Small Randomized Trials. Ann Surg 2021;273(3): 424–32.

48. AATS Wellness Committee, American Association for Thoracic Surgery website, Available at: https://www.aats.org/about-the-aats/committees/wellness-committee, (Accessed November 8, 2023), 2023.

49. Society of Thoracic Surgeons, Wellness Resources. Society of Thoracic Surgeons website. 2023, Available at: https://www.sts.org/resources/life-career/wellness-resources. Accessed November 8, 2023.

50. Cooke DT, Olive J, Godoy L, et al. The Importance of a Diverse Specialty: Introducing the STS Workforce on Diversity and Inclusion. Ann Thorac Surg 2019; 108(4):1000–5.

51. Trudell AM, Frankel WC, Luc JGY, et al. Enhancing Support for Women in Cardiothoracic Surgery Through Allyship and Targeted Initiatives. Ann Thorac Surg 2022;113:1676–83.
52. Williams KM, Hironaka CE, Wang H, et al. Women in Thoracic Surgery Scholarship: Impact on Career Path and Interest in Cardiothoracic Surgery. Ann Thorac Surg 2021;112:302–7.
53. Rangel EL, Castillo-Angeles M, Easter SR, et al. Incidence of Infertility and Pregnancy Complications in US Female Surgeons. JAMA Surg 2021. https://doi.org/10.1001/jamasurg.2021.3301.
54. Rangel EL, Smink DS, Castillo-Angeles M, et al. Pregnancy and motherhood during surgical training. JAMA Surg 2018;153(7):644–52.
55. Rangel EL, Castillo-Angeles M, Yung Hu Y, et al. Lack of Workplace Support for Obstetric Health Concerns is Associated with Major Pregnancy Complications: A National Study of US Female Surgeons. Ann Surg 2022. https://doi.org/10.1097/SLA.0000000000005550.
56. Wagner CM, Watt TMF, Ailawadi G, et al. Supporting Cardiothoracic Surgery Trainees Building Families: Creation of a Departmental Perinatal Policy. Ann Thorac Surg 2023. https://doi.org/10.1016/j.athoracsur.2023.07.001.
57. Pham DT, Stephens EH, Antonoff MB, et al. Birth trends and factors affecting childbearing among thoracic surgeons. Ann Thorac Surg 2014;98(3):890–5.
58. Leave of absence policy, American Board of Thoracic Surgery website, Available at: www.abts.org, (Accessed November 9, 2023), 2023.
59. Hu Y yung and BK. Surgical Education Culture Optimization through targeted interventions based on National comparative Data (SECOND) Trial, Available at: https://thesecondtrial.org. Accessed November 9, 2023.
60. Johnson HM, Torres MB, Möller MG, et al. Association of Women Surgeons' Comprehensive Initiative for Healthy Surgical Families during Residency and Fellowship Training. JAMA Surg 2023;158(3):310–5.
61. Song Y, Swendiman RA, Shannon AB, et al. Can We Coach Resilience? An Evaluation of Professional Resilience Coaching as a Well-Being Initiative for Surgical Interns. J Surg Educ 2020;77(6):1481–9.

Optimizing Work Relationships for Well-Being

Azzan N. Arif, MD[a],*, Aundrea Oliver, MD[b]

KEYWORDS

- Cardiothoracic surgery • Well-being • Workplace • Relationships • Interpersonal relationships
- Leadership • Teamwork • Communication

KEY POINTS

- The goals of this article are to identify common themes within the workplace that build relationships which can strengthen camaraderie, minimize burnout, and improve overall quality of patient care.
- Interpersonal relationships within the workplace directly affect the individual's ability and motivation to succeed. In our field of Cardiothoracic Surgery, the intensity of the work only magnifies professional interdependence.
- Different styles of leadership have been examined and shown to have an impact on team dynamics. While there is no correct method, a combination of styles, when used in the correct circumstance, allow the operating room team to excel.
- Psychological safety is another aspect of stability in the workplace. An unwelcoming environment that does not encourage communication in the workplace can lead to health care teams being unsatisfied in their positions.
- As surgeons we need the collective strength of our mid-level providers, physician colleagues in other disciplines, allied health professionals, nurses at every level, technicians, and administrative staff to become greater than just ourselves.

INTRODUCTION

Cardiothoracic Surgery has long been considered a demanding surgical specialty with high stress due to the complexity of the patients and the technical skills required to treat these patients. Cardiothoracic Surgery is often likened to aviation, given that errors in the field may lead to substantial harm and even mortality. Moreover, deficiencies in communication and suboptimal teamwork contribute to the errors in Cardiothoracic Surgery.[1] Optimizing well-being among cardiothoracic surgeons and their team through intentional team building, allows for improvements in patient care and overall job satisfaction.

The goals of this article are to identify common themes within the workplace that build relationships which can strengthen camaraderie, minimize burnout, and improve overall quality of patient care. Why is this important? A Harvard Business Review article found that our understanding of what leads to professional satisfaction is often misplaced. "While many of us strive for a meaningful job, an impressive title, or a sizable salary, we drastically undervalue the importance of interpersonal relationships, despite the extensive research showing that people, not the perfect job, lead to professional fulfillment."[2] Surveys involving people from a wide variety of industries and roles consistently reveal that individuals engaged in routine or

[a] Division of Thoracic Surgery, Department of Surgical Oncology, Fox Chase Cancer Center, Temple University Health Systems, 333 Cottman Avenue, Philadelphia, PA 19111, USA; [b] Department of Cardiovascular Sciences, East Carolina Heart Institute, East Carolina University, 115 Heart Drive, Greenville, NC 27834, USA
* Corresponding author.
E-mail address: Azzan.Arif@fccc.edu

Thorac Surg Clin 34 (2024) 261–269
https://doi.org/10.1016/j.thorsurg.2024.04.011
1547-4127/24/Published by Elsevier Inc.

challenging occupations can feel the same level of satisfaction and fulfillment as those in enjoyable or inspiring occupations. The key to this is to actively foster and cultivate relationships that are nurturing and instill a sense of purpose.[2] This highlights an important fact, who we work with and the roles they play are instrumental to a healthy and efficient workplace. This starts from the top, and leadership culture builds a framework for everyone to follow, either by example, or with thorough and thoughtful understanding of the team members' needs and conflicts.

M. Balch and colleagues highlighted the imperative of fostering a supportive workplace environment to mitigate stress and burnout among surgeons. The authors highlighted physician burnout often stems from an inefficient and potentially hostile work environment.[3] It is a widely held belief that surgical residencies are intensely challenging due to the hostile working environments shaped by the culture of surgery, which demands perfection and anything else is deemed a failure. The current surgical culture often does not reflect this lore, but within the specialty there are real and meaningful high stakes for our patients. Our field often attracts intense individuals who personally and professionally value excellence. This intensity is heightened by the long hours, sleepless nights, and considerable time away from family. These sacrifices only underscore the importance of nurturing healthy workplace relationships that positively impact our well-being and enable us to effectively lead our patient care teams.

IT STARTS WITH TEAMWORK AND COMMUNICATION

When researching what creates an optimal work environment for a treatment team, the common themes found are teamwork and communication. A review of the anesthesia literature underscores that health care is inherently interdisciplinary, requiring collaboration among physicians, nurses, and allied health professionals across varying specialties.[4] Effective teamwork plays a pivotal role in safeguarding patient care.[4,5] The literature indicates that the quality and safety of patient care may be compromised by insufficient coordination among health care providers at various organizational levels, resulting in issues such as delays in testing or treatment and conflicting information.[6,7] As is illustrated and emphasized in an editorial in Cardiac Surgery by Merry and colleagues,[8] the importance of teamwork and communication is critical for an interdisciplinary staff and conducive to safe patient care. Merry and colleagues also state that failures in communication and teamwork

are recurring contributors to adverse events in health care. A noteworthy discovery is the significance of minor events, when taken collectively, hold as much importance as major ones.[9-11] The Flawless Operative Cardiovascular Unified System (FOCUS) project is an initiative undertaken by the Society of Cardiovascular Anesthesiologists which is a multi-year study to learn and improve human errors in cardiac surgery. The goal is harm-free cardiac surgery. There is an added emphasis to the importance of fostering a work culture where staff feel not only comfortable but also are encouraged to speak up if they perceive any potential harm.[12,13] The errors they observed were categorized with evidence that improving teamwork and communication in health care can decrease human errors. Improving teamwork is an explicit objective of the WHO Surgical Safety Checklist.[14-16] What the WHO Surgical Safety Checklist has brought to every operating room is a form of direct communication among a team of members in order to prevent human error and remove never events.

Interpersonal relationships within the workplace directly affect the individual's ability and motivation to succeed. In our field of Cardiothoracic Surgery, the intensity of the work only magnifies professional interdependence. It starts with understanding the roles of the team and trusting one another. The American Association of Critical Care Nurses (AACN) has made noteworthy strides in creating guidelines for a healthy work environment (HWE). Their efforts have demonstrated that a conducive work environment correlates with increased engagement, reduced burnout, lower turnover rates, and enhanced patient care. Data from AACN reveal that units implementing the HWE standards outperformed those that did not. This includes enhancements in the overall health of the work environment, improved nurse staffing and retention, decreased moral distress, and a reduction in the incidence of workplace violence.[17] "The six standards illustrated included skilled communication, true collaboration, effective decision making, appropriate staffing, meaningful recognition, and authentic leadership."[17] Again, a common theme in their efforts included teamwork and communication.

Salas and colleagues proposed a model for teamwork that includes 5 dimensions: team orientation, team leadership, mutual performance monitoring, backup behavior, and adaptability.[18] These dimensions were supported by 3 coordinating factors: mutual trust, effective communication, and shared mental models within the team. The elegance of this model is 2 fold. The principles upon which the team is defined are clear, measurable, reproducible, and allow for room for growth. Adding to that platform, the "buy in" principles of the team that are based on goal alignment and group agreement. This allows for a team to encounter new challenges and respond in a coordinated and synergistic manner, deal with failure as a group with shared responsibility and accountability, and group innovation to allow for individual and group skill acquisition and professional growth. This makes room for personal growth at every level of the team and for every career level. If an individual believes that their performance matters and obtains group feedback of their importance to the success of that team, they are more likely to report a sense of fulfillment, meaning, and satisfaction. If an individual feels expendable, incapable, or abused, they are more likely to report significant dissatisfaction with their work environment, independent of their compensation or schedule. This personal perception is often rooted in the culture of the work environment and as we stated earlier that culture is framed by leadership. Therefore, it is prudent to understand the importance of leadership in the Cardiothoracic Surgery workplace.

THE EFFECT OF LEADERSHIP ON WORKPLACE RELATIONSHIPS

In the world of Cardiothoracic Surgery, the surgeon assumes the role of the pilot or conductor, guiding and orchestrating the operation alongside their team, each member playing a crucial role. Similar to the essential communication between a pilot and a co-pilot, the cardiothoracic anesthesiologist's contribution holds significant importance, as it directly influences the flow of the operation. As each respective professional leverages their medical and surgical expertise to treat the patient, the rest of the crew, including the nurses, surgical technicians, first-assists, allied professionals such as perfusionists, and trainees, attentively listen and act diligently in their roles. Direct communication is the key for each member on this team to execute their role at the highest level. Allowing everyone to feel empowered to voice concerns or seek clarification requires a blame-free and approachable environment. When the operation goes smoothly, the room flows like a beautiful symphony, but when emergent measures are required, this may not always be the case. Building and maintaining a culture of safety in the operating room will often dictate the patient's outcome. Similarly, developing and maintaining a "culture of safety" is common to all high-risk industries, including commercial aviation, the military, and health care.[1] This concept is grounded in research on organizations that "consistently minimize adverse events despite carrying out intrinsically complex and hazardous work."[1,19] Like the fields listed earlier, cardiothoracic surgery teams have a specific build in order to execute their tasks for each patient. Historically all recommendations and decisions made in the operating room must be granted by the surgeon as they will ultimately carry the responsibility of all outcomes. The stress this creates can lead to failure to realize the teamwork and communication necessary to arrive at the desired goal. Although similar in intensity and high stakes, there are measures built into the military unit, airplane cockpit, or nuclear power plant where human errors are expected and anticipated independent of leadership. This dyad of shared responsibility can mitigate portions of the unique stress of leadership and allow even those in charge to feel supported and valued.

Different styles of leadership have been examined and shown to have an impact on team dynamics. There is no one correct method but a combination of them that, when used in the correct circumstance, allow the operating room team to excel. It is not surprising that the leadership qualities of the attending surgeon will impact the function of the operating room team. As surgical team behavior has a direct impact on patient outcomes, exploring leadership styles has become an important aspect of surgical safety research.[1]

There are 2 prevalent leadership models: transactional and transformational leadership. Each model is discussed in terms of their applications and limitations. Transactional leaders, often likened to a commander, employ a leadership style built around rewards and punishments. They are responsible for assigning individual tasks, duties, and holding staff accountable. To encourage good performance, they use rewards in order to motivate their staff that translates to positive feedback in the operating room. This feedback becomes critical as it offers reassurance to each team member regarding their roles fostering a clear understanding of their responsibilities.[20] Transactional leadership is most effective in established systems where minimal change is required. Team members are familiar with their roles, and expectations are consistent allowing individuals to apply feedback to reach performance goals that are clearly defined.

In contrast, a transformational leadership style focuses on optimizing the team's abilities and efforts. Transformational leaders tend to exhibit 4 basic characteristics: inspiration, mobilization, morale, and conflict resolution. Inspiration involves the collaborative efforts of the team to explore alternatives that may better achieve the goal at hand, always prioritizing the greater good. Mobilization places importance on empowering efficient groups capable of completing tasks. This is executed by creating camaraderie and mutual interdependence among members who complement each other well. The third characteristic is morale, considered the most crucial attribute, as it involves boosting well-being and motivation within the team by establishing meaningful and enduring rapport between the team members. These characteristics position the leader as part of the team, empowering and holding the team accountable for any outcome, positive or negative. A common phrase used is "servant leader," which one who leads as a working member of the team often familiar with the roles they lead by personal experience. This leads to increase in morale for the whole team.[20] Lastly, transformational leaders excel at conflict resolution, allowing their team to maximize potential and capacity while minimizing friction. These leaders aim to constantly adapt and improve the system for the benefit of everyone, recognizing the team as a group of individuals with a common goal. For surgeons practicing transformational leadership, they encourage a democratic approach within their teams, supporting change for the greater good.[20]

Notably, each leadership style is dependent upon the task at hand, as more than one style of leadership from each model may be required for the best outcomes. Phenomenal leaders will usually ascertain qualities from both models in order to get the task done but at the same time foster an environment of cooperation and teamwork. In the context of building workplace relationships and well-being, a surgeon with a higher transformational leadership score was found to be exquisite at teamwork and communication. This observation has direct relevance to cardiac procedures, in which multiple specialties must work together. In a compelling study from the Harvard Business School published in 2003, researchers interviewed 16 cardiac surgical teams who were in the process of adopting minimally invasive cardiac procedures.[1,21] The findings revealed a strong correlation between the leadership style of the surgeon and a willingness of other operating room members to speak up. Teams with members who were willing to speak more freely were led by surgeons who "minimized power status rather than endorsed them."[22]

The leadership styles exhibited by the surgeons play a pivotal role in the well-being of their teams. A study investigating the association between leadership styles and well-being found that the transformational style of leadership contributed to an increase in quality of life and various outcome variables (extra effort, perceived leader effectiveness, and satisfaction) among nurses directly more than other leadership styles.[23] This is especially noteworthy, given the potential challenges between physicians and nurses. A study evaluating workplace conflict by measuring an institutional incident reporting system (IRS) found that 27.9% of the IRS were focused on interpersonal relationships, with the common incidents being negative emotion, disagreement, and interference.[24] What was interesting, and to some expected, was that 33% of those reports were from nurse–doctor interactions. Working in a conflicted workplace causes strain to an integral relationship, resulting in failure of communication, job dissatisfaction, and impairment of the efficacy of the treatment team.

The benefits of transformational leadership have been identified among surgeons and trainees in order for residents to craft their jobs. A study was conducted where surgeons who were considered transformational leaders by their residents were asked to practice 5 actions that would optimize job crafting in residents.[25] They would demonstrate positive behaviors of a proficient surgeon, allowing residents to progress with graduated autonomy, building personal professional relationships with the residents, and offering support when handling errors and complications, and lastly providing mentorship to residents with prioritizing competing interests. These actions led residents to feel more responsible in patient care, more constructive in relationships in the workplace, lowered workload stress and from surgical care duties, and less personal difficulties and errors in patient care. However, imbedded in this transformational leadership is the fundamental transactional leadership of surgery. When done well transactional leadership sets clear and consistent standards, goals, and feedback while delivering on promised incentives for high level team performance. Excellent surgeon leaders are more than inspirational, they can take discrete tasks and assign meaning and therefore value to them. They then translate that value from the task alone to individual team member worth and measured progress to a discrete goal accepted and valued by the entire team.

It is evident that building a healthy workplace environment in order to optimize well-being among team members requires strong leadership for the team to rely on and trust. Styles of leadership can differ at times but understanding workplace dynamics can reveal gaps in leadership needs that are critical to the health of the care team and ultimately the quality of care their patients receive. A strong leader is able to recognize those needs and pivot to draw upon the necessary strategy to stabilize and reinforce a balanced and productive workplace.

PSYCHOLOGICAL SAFETY AND ITS EFFECT ON WORKPLACE RELATIONSHIPS

The element of psychological safety represents another crucial factor influencing workplace relationships. When there is an aura of psychological safety in your working environment, teams are more likely to collectively believe they can take interpersonal risks. These risks can include but are not limited to speaking, posing questions, and sharing ideas.[26] This sense of psychological safety is directly related to enhanced workplace creativity, team learning, and team performance.[27] Despite the benefits listed, psychological safety has been lower across the health care field due to fear of speaking up, causing a commotion, or causing conflict. The solution came from leadership who valued changing culture.

An in situ interprofessional simulation performed at the Stanford University in their Department of Surgery attempting to improve teamwork and communication had identified a significant psychological barrier in communication. The study provided in situ simulations to health care professionals ranging from residents, attendings, and nursing. They found that a common barrier in communication in the operating room was due to hierarchical dynamics within OR staff. For instance, surgery and anesthesiology residents referred to their respective attendings as superiors and sometimes hesitated to communicate with others for fear of contradicting surgeons or anesthesiologists, individuals they felt were above them on the team hierarchy.[28] The other communication barrier faced was related to overall discouragement in communication among those staff members who were rude and unwelcoming members. These barriers introduced were key points of workplace relationships being hindered due to low psychological safety. On the other hand, when staff members were approachable and cordial, or when participants were in a simulation with familiar faces, there was less hesitation to communicate.

The inability to speak up is a significant issue that requires attention as it directly affects patient safety and their outcomes. Over 70% of adverse events were caused by behavior-related breakdowns in communication, according to the Joint Commission.[29] There have been measures undertaken to encourage psychological safety. The Department of Anesthesiology and Cardiothoracic Surgery at Barnes Jewish Hospital conducted a survey before and after implementing Team Strategies and Tools to Enhance Performance and Patient Safety (teamSTEPPS) training and the impact on perceived psychological safety. Their objectives were to improve psychological safety in the cardiothoracic operating rooms (CT ORs) encouraging all team members to speak up with concerns regarding safety issues, decreasing turnover, decreasing employee burnout, and improving error reporting. Although their results were not clinically significant, there was overall improvement in the outcomes they analyzed.[30]

Psychological safety is another aspect of stability in the workplace. An unwelcoming environment that does not encourage communication in the workplace can lead to health care teams that may feel less fulfillment in their positions. When team members feel safe and confident to speak up, it allows for better professional relationships among workplace members. What teamSTEPPS achieved was a system to encourage communication and provide a simulation exercise that enhances teamwork. This intervention is an example of a team recognizing a deficit in their teamwork that was imbedded in communication. Clear and direct strategy to address this deficit gave opportunity for shared goals and team member investment in culture shift at every level.

CONFLICT IN THE WORKPLACE

It is apparent that the key to building a healthy workplace environment requires a multidisciplinary approach that includes leadership support, communication, team building, and the ability to acknowledge and respond to conflict. In the stressful atmosphere of the field of surgery, it is the responsibility of all parties to buy in, allowing a haven for growth. What we have alluded to but have not delved into is conflict in the workplace and how this affects professional well-being.

The workplace environment of surgeons has long been perceived as intimidating, unwelcoming, fearsome, and threatening. Many a surgeon has regaled about a time in training when they were berated by an intimidating attending. In many circles it is seen as a rite of passage. This sentiment is not exclusive to surgeons, many nurses, surgical techs, perfusionists, and anesthesiologists may trade OR "war stories" as a similar badge of honor. In the worst of situations, poor and abusive leadership in the OR can create a culture of lateral violence, micro and macroaggressions as team members translate that behavior throughout the team hierarchy. A survey identifying prevalence of bullying among US surgeons found that reasons cited for bullying included stressful work, strict hierarchy, and a lack of institutional policy.[31] Barriers to reporting bullying included negative effects on career, reputation, and additional bullying. It was most prevalent among universities from male surgeons who were professors. Unabated, vindictive work environments can generate a toxicity that is typified by high staff turnover at all levels.

The consequences of harboring workplace interpersonal conflict have proven detrimental. In the realm of the nursing workforce, it has led to increased nurse turnover, which is costly to the workplace, not only in nominal value, but the greater problem is the loss of experienced nurses, resulting in an upsurge of nurse errors and patient mortality.[31] The opposite has also been shown, workplace compassion has decreased nurse turnover. Compassionate behavior also significantly affected psychological stress, which also dictated behavior and sleep quality.[32–34] Workplace interpersonal conflicts often arise due to miscommunication, stress, or unresolved competing priorities of tasks.[24] Such conflicts can cause disadvantageous effects on workers, including decrease in staff satisfaction and fulfillment, diminished team performance, and subsequently impact patients by leading to inefficient and poor patient care. These repercussions extend to increased rate of medical errors, increased burnout, and overall increased cost of care.

What can be done to resolve conflict efficiently within the workplace? First, instituting an adequate reporting system may provide an outlet for health care workers to express their concern and tackle interpersonal conflict. Incidental reporting systems have commonly been used for safety events, but reporting workplace conflict allows us to acknowledge and work to strengthen the interpersonal relationships among employees of the hospital.[24] Other measures have been taken to efficiently resolve conflict. For the past decade, the Royal College of Surgeons in Ireland delivered a transformative learning experience called "Professional Interactions" where junior residents in surgery and other acute care fields would gain the skills to better manage conflict and bullying.[33] The course focused on rational discourse, role playing, simulations, case studies, reflection exercises, and experience with critical incidents feedback. It simulated everyday workplace conflict and focused on how to address these stressful moments. The results from the course have received outstanding participant satisfaction. The practice of using simulations and involving all hospital staff allows an open environment for controlled conflict so that when it occurs in reality, one would be able to practice their newfound knowledge. As it is stated on examination prep, get it wrong now, so that you can get it right on the test.

Interpersonal conflict and poor communication in the workplace can lead to a stressful environment that increases turnover intention and burnout.[3,17,24,30,31,33] This provides an unsafe environment for patient care. This due to the failure of the 2 pillars of a healthy workplace environment—teamwork and communication. Conflict occurs because of poor communication and remains unresolved due to the same. As professionals we are to model the behavior we are seeking from our colleagues. The very weaknesses often cited about our field-intensity, high stakes, and high demand produce in us, the capacity to respond to conflict with the same strength and candor that we approach our surgical duties. Our ability to respect objective data, lean in to responsibility, and value excellence can translate into accountability based on truth and compassion that results in real and lasting change. As surgeons we need the collective strength of our mid-level providers, physician colleagues in other disciplines, allied health professionals, nurses at every level, technicians and administrative staff to become greater than just ourselves. Whatever we value most, toxicity, innovation, blind allegiance, excellence—it will dictate our culture and therefore the well-being of the team.

SUMMARY

We are privileged as health care workers to support the health of our communities, but it is our duty to influence a healthy workplace environment in order to optimize our professional well-being. In this article, we have learned the importance of trust and communication in the workplace. If there is proper communication and adequate teamwork, then we can minimize errors and improve patient outcomes. When there is structure in the operating room or on the wards, and everyone buys in, people feel fulfillment in their work and are motivated to work hard for the common objective. A safe culture that allows for growth and provides all team members a space to communicate their concerns helps all members feel like they matter. This series provides the framework by tackling important topics such as improving personal and professional wellness and minimizing burnout. It explores the roles of community involvement, both professional and personal, and the evolution of careers within our surgical specialty. The interplay of all these threads creates the safety net for our patients in the form of a well-functioning team. The physician leader can translate health and value or burnout and cynicism to the team, resulting in innovation and excellence or disintegration of a previously viable treatment team.

Leadership serves as the foundation to build and strengthen a culture of professional well-being. Though variations of leadership style have shown positive impact in certain circumstances, it is the combination of styles that provides the most optimal conditions for confidence and growth. Effective leadership entails the instinctive understanding of when change is imperative and when the continuation of successful practices is more beneficial. Leaders within the field bear the responsibility to tackle challenges such as psychological safety, professional well-being, and conflict resolution. It does not necessarily need to be the physician, as is evident by the excellent work from the AACN development of their HWE Standards. This dynamic and collaborative work at every level of the treatment team is integral to meaningful growth and improvement of the care we deliver as a team.

In conclusion, this article sets the stage for the future of health care. We are at the cusp of another great shift in medicine, and we have the opportunity to guide the direction of that shift. We have an opportunity to go beyond myopic self-absorption and personal gratification to understand the truest meaning of well-being. It is more than "well doing," "well getting," or "well reporting." It engages the best part of who we are, our humanity, and the humanity of the individuals we work alongside. The power of this togetherness allows us to harness all the talent of the team to provide the best and highest quality care for every patient we touch. Our ability to take on any deconstruction of our surgical past and upcycle our heritage as surgeons should propel us to become a better version of the giants before us. Not leaving go of the value of integrity, grit, excellence, and tenacity but adding to it an equally potent compassion and commitment to truth in the form of accountable leadership. Developing a healthy workplace environment brings structure to an institution and increases recruitment and retention at every level of the health care team. What we do today, and the culture we create now informs the next generation of health care providers. Let us give them a healthy head start.

CLINICS CARE POINTS

Pearls:

- Optimizing workplace well-being is best tackled by implementing strategies such as the WHO Surgical Safety Checklist and participating in initiatives like the FOCUS project.

These foundational pillars for effective teamwork and communication amplify patient safety and team camaraderie.

- Understanding and practicing different leadership styles positively impacts team dynamics and patient outcomes. Namely, fostering both transactional and transformational leadership qualities provides a culture of collaboration and innovation, leading to improved job satisfaction and patient care. Surgeons who exhibit mainly transformational qualities often invite a culture of teamwork where everyone feels their voice is heard and their mistakes are not scrutinized.

- Psychological safety is crucial in cultivating open communication and reducing workplace conflict. Interprofessional simulations aid health care teams in developing a hierarchical dynamic which encourages all members to have a voice and specify their concerns.

- Addressing workplace conflict using a structured reporting system and educational interventions help minimize the negative effects on team morale and patient care. Initiatives like the Royal College of Surgeons' "Professional interactions" program provide valuable tools for managing conflict and promoting a positive work environment.

Pitfalls:

- Failure to acknowledge the importance of building interpersonal relationships in professional fulfillment can lead to a culture that ignores teamwork and communication, leading to subpar patient care.

- Not addressing the hierarchical dynamics and provide an environment where members feel safe to speak up can lead to ineffective communication which ultimately can result in missed errors and compromising patient care.

- Ignoring conflict within the workplace can lead to a toxic work culture that leads to resentment and unhealthy team building. These unhealthy behaviors can influence increasing turnover, decreasing retention, and in turn decreasing the quality of patient care.

- Inconsistent leadership qualities can cause confusion among the team, hampering innovation and growth. It is important that leaders empower such qualities to provide healthy behaviors when tackling issues such as conflict, errors, and burnout.

DISCLOSURE

The authors have nothing to disclose.

REFERENCES

1. Wilson JL, Whyte RI, Gangadharan SP, et al. Teamwork and Communication Skills in Cardiothoracic Surgery. Ann Thorac Surg 2017;103(4):1049–54.
2. Rob C. To be happier at work, invest more in your relationships. Harvard Business Review. 2019. Available at: https://hbr.org/2019/07/to-be-happier-at-work-invest-more-in-your-relationships?ab=at_art_art_1x4_s03.
3. Balch CM, Freischlag JA, Shanafelt TD. Stress and Burnout Among Surgeons: Understanding and Managing the Syndrome and Avoiding the Adverse Consequences. Arch Surg 2009;144(4):371–6.
4. Manser T. Teamwork and patient safety in dynamic domains of healthcare: a review of the literature. Acta Anaesthesiol Scand 2009;53(2):143–51.
5. Kohn LT, Corrigan JM, Donaldson MS. To err is human: building a safer health system. Washington, DC: National Academy Press; 1999.
6. Baggs JG, Ryan SA, Phelps CE, et al. The association between interdisciplinary collaboration and patient outcomes in a medical intensive care unit. Heart Lung 1992;21:18–24.
7. Young GJ, Charns MP, Desai K, et al. Patterns of coordination and clinical outcomes: *a study of surgical services*. Health Serv Res 1998;33:1211–36.
8. Merry AF, Weller J, Mitchell SJ. Teamwork, communication, formula-one racing and the outcomes of cardiac surgery. J Extra Corpor Technol 2014;46(1):7–14.
9. de Leval MR, Carthey J, Wright DJ, et al. Human factors and cardiac surgery: A multicenter study. J Thorac Cardiovasc Surg 2000;119:661–72.
10. Solis-Trapala IL, Carthey J, Farewell VT, et al. Dynamic modelling in a study of surgical error management. Stat Med 2007;26:5189–202.
11. Mishra A, Catchpole K, McCulloch P. The Oxford NOTECHS System: Reliability and validity of a tool for measuring teamwork behaviour in the operating theatre. Qual Saf Health Care 2009;18:104–8.
12. Martinez EA, Thompson DA, Errett NA, et al. High stakes and high risk: A focused qualitative review of hazards during cardiac surgery. Anesth Analg 2011;112:1061–74.
13. Gurses AP, Kim G, Martinez EA, et al. Identifying and categorising patient safety hazards in cardiovascular operating rooms using an interdisciplinary approach: A multisite study. BMJ Qual Saf 2012;21:810–8.
14. Haynes AB, Weiser TG, Berry WR, et al. A surgical safety checklist to reduce morbidity and mortality in a global population. N Engl J Med 2009;360:491–9.
15. Neily J, Mills PD, Young-Xu Y, et al. Association between implementation of a medical team training program and surgical mortality. JAMA 2010;304:1693–700.
16. de Vries EN, Prins HA, Crolla RMPH, et al. Effect of a comprehensive surgical safety system on patient outcomes. N Engl J Med 2010;363:1928–37.
17. Ulrich Beth, Cassidy Linda, Barden Connie, et al. National Nurse Work Environments - October 2021: A Status Report. Crit Care Nurse 2022;42(5):58–70.
18. Salas E, Sims D, Burke C. Is there a "Big Five" in teamwork? Small Group Res 2005;36:555–99.
19. Patient Safety Primer: safety culture. Available at: https://psnet.ahrq.gov/primers/primer/5/safety-culture. [Accessed 8 November 2016].
20. Arnold D, Fleshman JW. Leadership in the Setting of the Operating Room Surgical Team. Clin Colon Rectal Surg 2020;33(4):191–4.
21. Edmondson AC. Speaking up in the operating room: how team leaders promote learning in interdisciplinary action teams. J Manag Stud 2003;40:1419–52.
22. Yule S, Flin R, Paterson-Brown S, et al. Non-technical skills for surgeons in the operating room: a review of the literature. Surgery 2006;139:140–9.
23. Sabbah IM, Ibrahim TT, Khamis RH, et al. The association of leadership styles and nurses well-being: a cross-sectional study in healthcare settings. Pan Afr Med J 2020;36:328.
24. Jerng JS, Huang SF, Liang HW, et al. Workplace interpersonal conflicts among the healthcare workers: Retrospective exploration from the institutional incident reporting system of a university-affiliated medical center. PLoS One 2017;12(2):e0171696.
25. Domínguez LC, Dolmans D, Restrepo J, et al. How Surgical Leaders Transform Their Residents to Craft Their Jobs: Surgeons' Perspective. J Surg Res 2021;265:233–44.
26. Edmondson A. Psychological safety and learning behavior in work teams Amy Edmondson. Adm Sci Q 1999;44:350–83.
27. O'donovan R, Mcauliffe E. A systematic review of factors that enable psychological safety in healthcare teams. Int J Qual Health Care 2020;32(4):240–50.
28. Shi R, Marin-Nevarez P, Hasty B, et al. Operating Room In Situ Interprofessional Simulation for Improving Communication and Teamwork. J Surg Res 2021;260:237–44.
29. JCAHO. Sentinel event statistics. Hospital authority Hong Kong: Annual report on sentinel events; 2007.
30. Ridley CH, Al-Hammadi N, Maniar HS, et al. Building a Collaborative Culture: Focus on Psychological Safety and Error Reporting. Ann Thorac Surg 2021;111(2):683–9.
31. Pei KY, Hafler J, Alseidi A, et al. National Assessment of Workplace Bullying Among Academic Surgeons in the US. JAMA Surg 2020;155(6):524–6.

32. Wang T, Abrantes ACM, Liu Y. Intensive care units nurses' burnout, organizational commitment, turnover intention and hospital workplace violence: A cross-sectional study. Nurs Open 2023;10(2):1102–15.

33. Zhang SE, Liu W, Wang J, et al. Impact of workplace violence and compassionate behaviour in hospitals on stress, sleep quality and subjective health status among Chinese nurses: a cross-sectional survey. BMJ Open 2018;8(10):e019373.

34. O'Keeffe DA, Brennan SR, Doherty EM. Resident Training for Successful Professional Interactions. J Surg Educ 2022;79(1):107–11.

Personal Relationships and Well-being for Cardiothoracic Surgeons

Jamie Dickey Ungerleider, MSW, PhD[a],*,
Korie Candis Jones-Ungerleider, MD[b], Graham Dickey Ungerleider, MD[a,2],
Ross M. Ungerleider, MD, MBA[a,1]

KEYWORDS

- Cardiothoracic surgery • Well-being • Teamwork • Relationship skills • Burnout

KEY POINTS

- Relationship science over the past 40 years has brought to light the significance of secure, connected and stable relationships in our lives.
- We are verbs, not nouns. Nouns are labels and static and do not permit change. You are constantly growing. You are not stuck and doomed to always be whatever label someone decides to place on you.
- Accepting influence from others (both at work and at home) helps to build strong partnerships. When there is a failure to accept influence, relationships tend to fail.
- One of the most powerful tools for building strong relationships is the ability to make and accept repair attempts.

INTRODUCTION AND SUMMARY OF RESEARCH

As surgeons, and as providers of surgical care, we are often taught about leadership, and there is no question that surgeons need to be able to *take charge* and lead. We also learn a lot about "followership" and depending on the circumstances and where we are on the hierarchy of knowledge or authority, we can be pretty good at *taking orders* and following someone's lead.

What we do not learn much about is *partnering*, yet it is the ability to partner that creates the mortar that holds together the bricks of our relationships both at work and at home.

This article is devoted to the art of partnering by cardio thoracic (CT) surgeons, particularly with their significant others/spouses and family members, although the science behind the skills and practices that we will present can lead to improved partnering in the professional setting as well and can result in more secure and successful relationships at both home and at work.

The challenge of partnering by CT surgeons with their spouses and significant others is real, and it is measurable. It is very likely connected to the incidence of burnout and work-related distress among CT surgeons that has resulted in their withdrawal from engagement and decreased satisfaction with their professional lives. In a study published by the American Association for Thoracic Surgery (AATS) well-being committee in 2022,[1] a majority of CT surgeons reported being moderately to severely physically and emotionally

[a] Institute for Integrated Life Skills, LLC., 431 Riverbend Drive, Advance, NC 27006, USA; [b] Division of Cardiac Surgery, University of Michigan Medical Center, Ann Arbor, MI, USA
[1] Present address: 431 Riverbend Drive, Advance, NC 27006.
[2] Present address: 1766 Fulmer Street, Ann Arbor, MI 48104.
* Corresponding author. 431 Riverbend Drive, Bermuda Run, NC 27006.
E-mail address: jamieungerleider@icloud.com

Thorac Surg Clin 34 (2024) 271–280
https://doi.org/10.1016/j.thorsurg.2024.04.008
1547-4127/24/© 2024 Elsevier Inc. All rights reserved.

exhausted at work, feeling a sense of dread when thinking about work, and having a lack of enthusiasm when thinking about work.

The impact of this work-related burnout has an undeniable influence on all aspects of the lives of many surgeons. In a recent report generated by the well-being committee for the AATS and presented at the AATS 2023 annual meeting,[2] 66% of respondents to a survey sent to the significant others and spouses of CT surgeons felt that burnout was having a moderate-to-severe impact on the lives of their CT surgeon partners, and this was particularly true for those spouses or significant others who surgeon partners worked longer hours (68.4 vs 60.4 h/wk; $P = .005$). Even at the preferred commitment of 60 h/wk, CT surgeons are working an additional.5 Full - time employment (FTE) compared to the more typical US worker's 40 hour work per week! The significance of work hours on the family is even more evident in the response of 63% of spouses and significant others who felt that their CT surgeon partner's schedule did not leave enough time for family life. This finding was overwhelmingly related to work hours. Those spouses and significant others who agreed that there was no time for family life have CT surgeon partners who work more than 40 h/wk *more* than those spouses and significant others who felt the schedule did leave adequate time for family life (70 vs 48.6 h/wk; $P < .001$).

The effect of this on the lives of CT surgeons is predictable. Spouses and significant others of CT surgeons found that their partners had less empathy (42%), were less connected to loved ones (48%), had less interest in social activities (54%), and less connected to outside interests and hobbies (57%). All of this was most significant for those partners who had children aged under 19 years living in the home, which is a likely contributor to stress. However, when children are exposed to a stressed relationship, they often have little ability to understand the reasons for the stress and may even believe that they are the cause of it.

In this same study, spouses and significant others reported that they rarely had calm, good-natured interactions with their surgeon partner (23%), that they rarely engaged in activities together (40%), that they did not spend a healthy amount of time together (48%) and most disturbingly, that they could not find enough time for intimacy (52%). This hardly depicts the type of relationships that these couples hoped for when they embarked on their life journey together.

Relationship research over the past 40 years has brought to light the significance of secure, connected, and stable relationships in our lives. The Harvard Longitudinal Study of Adult Development is one of the most famous longitudinal studies ever performed. It tracked the lives of 724 men for over 80 years. One group was a cohort of sophomores at Harvard. The other group consisted of boys from Boston's poorest neighborhoods in the 1930s. After initial interviews and medical testing, their lives were followed over several decades. The study had 4 directors in order to keep it going over the years. Some of the boys ascended the ladder of success and some went in the opposite direction. Many are still alive and some of the findings are presented in a recent book[3] by the current director of the study. The lessons from the tens of thousands of pages of information generated from these lives point unequivocally to one common element that was present in the lives of those who achieved happy lives, and it was not wealth, fame, or a commitment to hard work. The clearest lesson simply stated is that good relationships keep us happier and healthier.

A second important study that underscores the importance of relationships was performed by James Coan.[4] He put people into MRI scanners, and then he delivered small electric shocks to them. When they got the shock, the parts of their brains that indicate stress lit up like a Christmas tree. Then, he had them hold the hands of others including strangers and spouses. When they held the hand of those with whom they were in a meaningful, trusting relationship, the shock had less of an effect, both as demonstrated on the MRI, as well as to how the shock was perceived by the subject. He then studied the hand holders and amazingly, it appeared that the shock was shared—distributed between 2 brains. By either literally (in our relationships at home) or metaphorically (in our work relationships) holding the hands of our partners, we can diminish the allostatic load of the stress from our challenges. This is why strong relationships keep us happy and healthy.

We learn about relationships early in life. Research by John Bowlby, Mary Ainsworth, Mary Main, Eric Hesse, Dan Siegel, and others[5,6] emphasizes the impact that our relationships with our early caretakers have on our sense of security in the world in childhood and throughout our lives. In addition to our basic biological needs for food and shelter, we all need a secure base to which we belong. While we can develop secure relationships as adults, even if we did not have secure relationships with our parents, it requires intention and the re-experiencing of relationships, which are safe, secure, competent, compassionate, consistent, and caring with significant others. Ideally, we have these relationships with our parents and extended family from birth and throughout childhood and thankfully, it is never too late to engage in these relationships because it is through these relationships that we internalize a sense of security and of being loved for who we truly are, long before we begin to erroneously define our value by our accomplishments, titles, or other external reflections that we think distinguish us such as the car we drive, the home we live in, or who we know. It is through our relationships with parents and other adults who are in the role of caretaker or teacher that we learn to self-regulate and manage our responses to life's demands. Depending on the nature of these relationships, some familiar patterns of relating to ourselves or to others may emerge. Some examples of these patterns are (1) learning not to trust others in relationships, (2) competing against others for recognition, (3) expecting one's self to be perfect with a loud internal (and external) critic when there is a failure, (4) acting out in frustration and anger due to an inability to self-soothe when needs are not being met, and (5) finding other avenues rather than relationships to create security/stability in life.[7] As human beings, we as a species are wired in a way that makes us very sensitive to rejection. When a sense of security, epistemic trust, and a sense of belonging are not experienced in our early years, we are vulnerable to developing an intense fear of not belonging and being accepted, creating a shame cycle of trying to not acknowledge that we have needs and then having shame when we do have them or when we fail to perform to the perfection that we believe is needed in order to be loved. We never outgrow the need for supportive and secure relationships with others to help us regulate our emotions, especially during times of stress.[8–10]

Turning Toward, Against, or Away

Research on relationships at all levels of development suggests that 1 of 3 things are happening in our relationships at any given time.

1) We *turn toward*, and the person in the relationship feels seen, understood, and secure/soothed in the warmth, stability, and belonging of the relationship. Turning toward invites authenticity and generates trust without the fear of judgment, criticism, or shame and also without the fear of abandonment or loss of belonging. John Gottman describes this as a *friend* relationship,[11,12] and Dan Wile characterizes this as creating a cycle of *empathy*.[13,14] As mentioned earlier, we learn this ability to *turn toward* from our relationship with our primary caregivers.[8] When we feel truly seen, understood, and soothed as children, then we cultivate an internalized capacity to regulate our emotions and explore our beliefs with curiosity.

We extend this *Curiosity, Openness, Acceptance,* and *Loving-kindness* not only to ourselves but also to others we encounter as we seek to manage the demands of our lives. Dan Siegel describes this as practicing COAL. Worthiness is not attached to performance or to having to fit in or to meet expectations. Conversations are centered around trying to explore and understand another so that their perspectives can be heard and valued. Most of us would like to be seen, heard, understood, and valued.

2) We *turn against*, and the person in the relationship feels judged, criticized, and possibly shamed for not meeting expectations. Gottman has described this as an *enemy* relationship, and Dan Wile suggests that it creates an *adversarial* cycle. The message is that the person (whether ourselves or another) is defective and unworthy of belonging unless they change to fit-in with expectations. As with turning toward, turning against is often learned through our relationship with our primary caregivers. When we grow up feeling judged, criticized, shamed, and even being punished if we fail to perform or achieve perfection, we are at risk for both internalizing this loud critical voice as well as for extending it to others. There is a loss of curiosity and exploration in order to understand and join with compassion. The relationship, whether with others or with ourselves, ceases to be one of soothing (emotional regulation) and understanding. A consequence of this is that it accelerates fear and anxiety from the worry that we will not be "good enough" if we do not achieve perfection or meet expectations. It is difficult to grow, change, and reach our potential when in the dysregulating grip of fear and anxiety related to our worthiness. In the adversarial cycle, we turn against others or ourselves with criticism or judgment when we are irritated or disappointed with a behavior or outcome from an event. The adversarial (enemy) cycle is also characterized by a tendency to put problems, when they exist, inside the other person and then blame them for their inadequacy. Interactions are organized around interrogating, judging, and fixing. Most people do not want to be interrogated, judged, and fixed.

3) We *turn away*, and the person in the relationship feels alone and abandoned. Gottman describes this as a *stranger* relationship, and Dan Wile characterizes it as creating a cycle of *withdrawal*. The message is that it is not safe to see others or even oneself in their (our) entirety. There is often a false belief that accompanies turning away that if we do not look at the parts

of others or ourselves, we judge as inferior or unworthy of love, they will not exist and will not need to be acknowledged or processed. Even though we may exile these parts, they are still there. Turning away may evolve when we learn in our relationship with our primary caregivers that relationships are not important and they can be messy, take too much energy, and cannot provide the feeling of belonging and acceptance that is more likely to be attached to accomplishment and performance. Unlike turning toward or turning against, where relationships have energy (regulated or dysregulated), turning away creates a false sense of emotional regulation as we disengage from needs (ours or those of others) and the valuing of the relationship and its importance. A consequence of this is loss of the ability to be intimate and genuine with oneself or with others. In highly stressful medical fields, like cardiothoracic surgery, this can contribute to depersonalization (inability to have a relationship with self or with others) and result in the syndrome of burnout. In the withdrawal cycle, we turn away or withdraw from others or ourselves with dismissiveness when needs are overwhelming, behaviors do not meet our expectations, or we experience the person or situation as being unworthy of our attention or too time consuming to manage. Individuals with this style of relating often have a strategy that includes dismissiveness of feelings. Turning away can also look like trying to control relationships through micromanaging in ways to keep them from getting too close, vulnerable, or demanding.

And just to be clear again, we do this with ourselves as much as we do this with others.

We are enemies to ourselves when we have a loud internal critic.

We are strangers to ourselves when we tend to ignore our feelings.

We are friends to ourselves when we cultivate curiosity and loving self-compassion.

The Importance of Early Relationships

Research on human attachment (what we learned about security and trust associated with relationships from our early primary care givers) suggests that what we experienced in these earliest relationships *between* ourselves and important others ultimately manifests in our relationships *within* our self.[5,6] Expanding on terminology introduced by Stan Tatkin,[15] those who turn away from themselves and others become *islands*—at risk for depersonalization (disconnecting from their feeling

self as they treat themselves or others more like a machine or an object) since relationships are not seen as an important source of understanding and soothing. For islands, tasks, achievement and reaching goals supersede relationships and connecting. Islands manage their insecurities, fears, and worries by trying to avoid feelings and relationships that invite them to experience vulnerability. They frequently put tasks, goals, and accomplishments ahead of relationships and attempt to not engage with or to expect those with whom they are in relationship not to invite vulnerability or have many needs. Islands tend to view others as commodities, and they expect high achievement and performance from those with whom they are close. Those who turn against themselves and others become like *waves*— desiring relationships, often idealizing what the relationship can provide, and then receding from their "shore" when that idealized relationship "disappoints" due to the imperfection that is inherent in all humans. Waves may have experienced parents who were sometimes available and sometimes not. Because of this inconsistency, they may have trouble trusting others in relationships. Like the metaphor of the wave, they yearn for connection and tend to idealize others only to crash and feel frustration and anger when they realize that the other person is a fallible human being. Waves can be very volatile in their relationships and have difficulty self-soothing. Additionally, waves may shape shift who they are depending on the circumstances and in doing so, not be true to who they are authentically. This can be confusing and also take a toll on others, as it is hard to know who will show up.[15]

Both of these relationship styles can predispose us to struggle, dissatisfaction, and burnout. In essence, islands manage their emotions by trying not to have them and waves manage their emotions by hoping others will make everything *ok*, and then blaming them when they cannot.

Then there are those who turn toward themselves and others—*anchored* with compassion and forgiveness for themselves and others as they find the courage to see and accept what is present without judgment, to learn, to love, and to accept struggle in themselves and in others. Research would suggest our relationship style characterizes how we lead, work, and survive or thrive during times of challenge.[16]

Take a moment to reflect on your preferred approach to relationships—particularly the one with yourself. Do you prefer being an island (relationships are secondary to achievement), a wave (relationships are desired and I tend to put that person on a pedestal, but am often left feeling disappointed in them, or myself, when they (or I) fail to be perfect), or have you learned to be an anchor (relationships take work, forgiveness, courage, and compassion and are an important part of your life)?

Over the years, we have learned a lot about the importance of having secure, connected, compassionate, curious, competent, consistent, and caring relationships in our lives, and there are many similarities between what we needed as children from our parents and what we need from our partners in committed relationships as adults. Throughout our lives we need to feel seen, heard, understood, and valued. In the best of circumstances, this happens from birth throughout childhood and on into our adult lives; however, not everyone has this experience, and the good news is that it does not have to determine the trajectory of future relationships. If we are willing and open to learn and to grow, we can establish an internal sense of security through treating ourselves as worthy of dignity and belonging no matter the external conditions or accomplishments of our life. Similarly, we can choose relationships that mirror our dignity and worthiness to belong that are not based on any external criteria. The good news is that even if we did not grow up in a family with these qualities of being seen, heard, understood, and valued, we can learn to create them later in life and not repeat the disappointing experiences of the past. Some have used the metaphor of an anchor to describe this relationship with our self and others because it is from a secure sense of self and a secure base with others that we are mostly likely to learn, grow, and reach our potential. Just as the metaphor of the anchor, which is able to withstand the storms of life and stay securely grounded, when we have our own internal sense of security and of being grounded, we are able to withstand the difficulties and problems of life with greater equanimity.[8]

We cannot help but exchange energy and information with those around us, and those who are closest to us are the ones who are most deeply impacted.[17] Imagine the significant other of a CT surgeon looking forward to a date night, a vacation, or to share a birthday celebration with their partner only to have plans canceled at the last minute due to an unanticipated clinical emergency. Although the partner of the surgeon logically understands the importance of the clinical event, they may get physiologically activated by the experience especially if it has been a frequent event. We are all especially susceptible to this type of activation if we have had previous experiences with rejection or not being able to influence and manage experiences that are important to us. The spouse or significant other may choose to withdraw or become frustrated and irritated as a way of protecting themselves. And, what about the surgeon, who is exhausted and who was equally looking forward to the planned event and who finally gets to come home in anticipation of being welcomed, only to find their spouse or significant other has turned away and is unavailable or who is turning against and exhibiting frustration, irritation, or anger? How will the surgeon not feel rejected or blamed in return? Ideally, the surgeon and their partner would turn toward one another and notice their disappointment at not being able to have the experience they both wanted. They would listen deeply, provide reassurance, and try to brainstorm some different solutions or perhaps get a coach or counselor to provide support for their relationship. We cannot help but be impacted by the people and environments in which we spend our time. Knowledge of this helps us develop awareness of the importance of providing compassionate support to ourselves, our partners and children, as well as seeking outside support when we lack the tools and skills to do this and are living in unsupportive environments.

In the remainder of this article, we will provide some evidence-based suggestions for turning toward your significant others, children, and other family members in order to cultivate more secure and satisfying relationships.

Tools for Improving Relationships

Commitment and attunement

Secure relationships are built on a core of attunement and trust. Attunement resides in the ability to be mindfully aware of *yourself*, of *others*, and of *context*. The neurologic basis for this is beautifully described by Dan Siegel in his book, *Mindsight*.[18] Attunement, when it exists for a relationship (whether among work team members, or the important others you relate to), is connected to our yearning to feel seen, heard, understood, and valued. Which is ultimately connected to our need to feel safe and secure. Which, in turn, is connected to our very real and basic need to belong. There are techniques that can be learned and practiced for cultivating cultures of attunement. In most cases, you will need to turn off your automatic patterns of relating, particularly if you lean toward being an island or a wave. Attunement, at its core, generates *trust*. I see you, hear you, and value you. In his book on the science of trust,[12] John Gottman emphasizes the importance of commitment, and ultimately, it is through commitment that many couples (or team members) find a way to hang together even when times are difficult. Perhaps, especially when times are difficult. People who spend the time and energy to see, hear, understand, and value each other (who are attuned to one another) and who send a message of commitment—"I will be there for you. I will come when you call me, and I will stand by you when you need me"—make relationships work. Contrast that concept to the often-repeated failures of commitment, particularly in the world of CT surgery, when a failure or struggle invites a turning away or turning against an individual, often to the extent of replacing or diminishing them. When you meet a couple who have been together for decades, ask them about times that their commitment was the glue that got them through some challenges. They will all have stories to share.

We all yearn to feel a sense of safety, security, trust, and belonging with those most significant to us. We often experience this when we ourselves feel truly seen, heard, understood, and valued by those closest to us. Therefore, the first step in any interaction is to first attune to ourselves and secondly to the other person.

There are numerous ways to attune to oneself. They generally include pausing and noticing our inward state. We all have a window of tolerance, which is a metaphor for how well we are internally regulated at any given moment (**Fig. 1**). At the top of the window is our sympathetic response or fight/flight response and at the bottom of the window is our parasympathetic response of shutting down or fainting. Before we attune to another person, we need to check-in with ourselves and notice our own state of regulation or dysregulation and self-soothe through breathing, reflection, or some other activity that invites us to be at ease with ourselves before connecting and attuning to another. Additionally, we need to explore our own mind through attuning and reflecting so that we have greater awareness of our own thoughts, beliefs, feelings, hopes, and expectations. In other words,

we want to explore our internal world through seeing, hearing, understanding, and valuing our own self and our needs and perspectives.

Once we have attuned to ourselves, we can then explore, from a stable core of self-awareness, to learn more about the experiences, beliefs, feelings, thoughts, and hopes of another person with whom we are in a relationship. In other words, we convey a sense of valuing their perspective with curiosity, openness, and acceptance of both our differences and similarities. We turn toward them to explore, understand, and join them. As an aside, when we use the term, "join," we do not necessarily mean that we agree with the other person, although we may. Rather, we join them by having them feel seen, heard, understood and valued, and supported by our genuine curiosity, kindness, and acceptance of what is real for them.

Attunement can also look like a bid for connection or an expression of a desire to spend time with another in a way that lets the other know that they are a source of delight and joy in our lives and not an obligation or responsibility.

Attunement to another requires an open, curious, and learning mindset.[19] We have to let go of knowing and thinking we are right as we open ourselves to the possibilities contained within another person's perspectives, especially when their perspectives are different from our own. It is important to remember that 2 people can have very different experiences of the same thing.[20] Unless we ask the other person and find ways to share with one another, we may never know that we are having different experiences of the same event. This is nicely depicted by the image shown in **Fig. 2**.[21] As you look at this image, you may be sure that you are seeing a dress that is a certain color and your certainty creates for you an expectation that everyone else sees the same thing. However, it turns out that some people see this

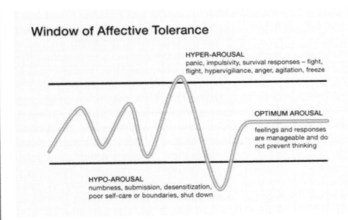

Window of Affective Tolerance

HYPER-AROUSAL
panic, impulsivity, survival responses – fight, flight, hypervigilance, anger, agitation, freeze

OPTIMUM AROUSAL
feelings and responses are manageable and do not prevent thinking

HYPO-AROUSAL
numbness, submission, desensitization, poor self-care or boundaries, shut down

Fig. 1. The affective window of tolerance defines the zone in which we are resourced to respond to stress or challenge. When an individual goes out the top of the window of tolerance, it is typically a fight/flight response and characterized by fear, anger, or loss of emotional regulation—typically a sympathetic nervous system response. When someone goes out the bottom of the window, it is typically a freeze or shutdown—a parasympathetic response. The window of tolerance is dynamic and can be enlarged by increasing ones internal and external resources.

Safe and secure relationships are fostered by commitment and attunement, which is manifested as mindful honoring and valuing of others so that they feel seen, heard, understood, valued, and safe. This safety nurtures intimacy (and in organizations, intimacy is expressed as respectful understanding and accepting of differences as factors that enhance and not detract from the capability of the team). Furthermore, when commitment is trusted, the environment becomes one in which it is safe for individuals to be the most authentic expressions of their feelings, beliefs, perspectives, and values. And these are the relationships that grow and thrive over time. Secure and safe relationships do not flourish in a culture of dismissiveness (turning away) or derisiveness (turning against).

Accepting influence

In his interview with the Harvard Business Review several years ago, John Gottman suggested that accepting influence can be one of the most powerful tools you can learn for cultivating a strong partnership.[24] We all need to allow ourselves to be influenced by those with whom we are in important and meaningful relationships. When we are willing to try new experiences or are willing to experiment with, share or try-on a differing perspective, we send a message to our important others that they and their needs and perspectives matter and are valuable. Imagine having a salt shaker but instead of it being full of salt, imagine that it is full of "yeses." And you can sprinkle them around in your relationships. "Yes," that sounds like a good idea. "Yes," tell me more. I have not thought of it that way before. "Yes," if that is important to you, then I will do it. "Yes, Yes, Yes." As opposed to "No." Does not the word "No" even create a different feeling in your body? Notice it. "No," we do not do things that way around here. "No," I do not need your ideas. "No," we will not do that. Not now. Not ever. "No," there is no way that dress is white and gold (or blue and black)!

Accepting influence can be promoted by a practice of being curious and open (the first part of COAL—Curious, Open, Accepting, with Loving kindness),[25] which expands upon and elevates accepting influence to a partnering of understanding by encouraging us to adopt a learning as opposed to a knowing mindset.

We are *verbs*—constantly evolving and growing because of our ability to influence and be influenced by each other. We are not *nouns*—labels doomed to be stuck forever by the descriptor someone decides to stick on us.

And this is challenging because we all work simultaneously with 2 different types of systems:

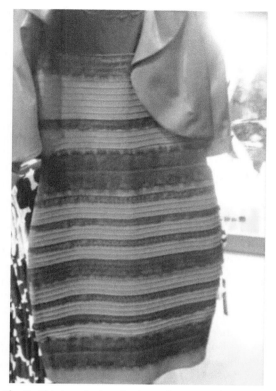

Fig. 2. This is a photo of a dress. Some people see this dress as blue and black, others as white and gold. If you assumed someone was having the same experience as you, you might be wrong, unless you checked it out. And who is right? We can have different experiences of the same thing. (*From*: McRaney D, How Minds Change: The Surprising Science of Belief, Opinion and Persuasion. 2022, New York. Portfolio / Penguin).

dress as blue and black while others are convinced it is white and gold. Who is right? And more importantly, if you did not explore in an open-minded way to learn about the perspectives of another, you might never know that others might be having a very different experience than you of this "same thing."

In cultures of commitment and attunement, individuals are permitted to embrace the *5 freedoms* as described by Virginia Satir[7]: The freedoms to (1) see and hear what is here instead of what should be, was, or will be; (2) say what one feels and thinks instead of what one should; (3) feel what one feels instead of what one ought; (4) ask for what one wants, instead of always waiting for permission; and (5) take risks on one's own behalf instead of choosing to be only "secure" and not rock the boat. This last freedom is also a key element in systems and relationships that are psychologically safe.[22,23]

mechanical and complex adaptive (which includes the biologically driven system of relationships).

A mechanical system might be something like a ventilator, or an airplane. We expect them to perform in a predictable and reliable manner. They lend themselves to checklists and protocols to enhance reproducibility. They are not supposed to exhibit emergent (novel, innovative, and unexpected) behaviors,[a] and if they do, we generally bring in a repair person who interrogates, judges, and fixes them in order to get them to conform to expectations for their performance. Most of us do not want to be interrogated, judged, and fixed. Mechanical systems lend themselves to task orientation—we do not have a relationship with mechanical systems.

Complex adaptive systems (which include the biological systems that are humans and the relationships between us) are unpredictable and variable. They lend themselves to curiosity and openness to possibilities and emergent behavior is welcomed. When there are problems, we explore to understand and join. Most of us, when there are challenges would like to be understood. Complex adaptive systems lend themselves to relationship orientation and a partnership approach. For a partnership to be strong, we need to learn to be curious, not judgmental.

The ability to be curious is emphasized by the dilemma of the cube[7,26] (Fig. 3). Imagine a box and inside that box is a cone—like the ones you see in parking lots or highways. And imagine that the box has 2 peepholes. Someone looking through peephole A, at the side, might see something like a triangle, and someone looking through peephole A on the top might see a circle.

Who is right? The (what we like to call) Capital T TRUTH is the consensus of perspectives.

In a *yes* culture, where we are attuned to others and give them the freedoms to see what they really see, we are curious and willing to accept their input, and we invite descriptions of what they see.

Adopting a learning versus knowing mindset

Strong and secure partnering requires a mindset that is willing to not know and be willing to struggle and occasionally fail. Part of learning, relevant to partnering, is to be open to exploring how to be influenced by others. Knowing—unfortunately too well engrained in our medical culture—embraces an attitude that differentiates us into experts, who are supposed to know everything, and the rest of us, who do not. We are either smart or we

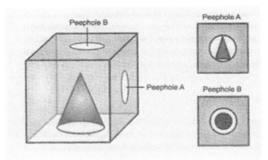

Fig. 3. The dilemma of the cube demonstrates how people can become convinced of that what they are seeing is the truth when, in fact, it may only be a part of the truth. The *whole truth* is the consensus of perspectives. (*From:* Ungerleider RM, Ungerleider JD, Strand A: Discovering Your Mindful Heart: An Explorer's Guide. Developing your internal resources to manage life's demands. 2020, Indianapolis, IN: Balboa Press).

are not. In her work studying 10 year olds who were either praised for being hard workers who were willing to see their limitations and to constantly learn, or for being validated as smart, Carol Dweck[19] found that those children who embraced learning showed significant improvement in performance over time, whereas those praised for being smart actually regressed and saw a 20% decrement in their performance over time. The point is, in a partnership, we are likely to be more successful if we do not approach our partners as if we are the knowers and they are our checklists. That is not a recipe for long-term strong partnerships.

Making and accepting repair attempts

Finally, no matter how hard we try and how much we learn, none of us operates from a secure base of connection, compassion, curiosity, competence, consistency, and openness at all times. We all have our moments of responding as an island or a wave. In research on couple relationships and relationships between parents and children, it has been found repeatedly that it is often not the rupture itself, but rather how that rupture is repaired that makes all the difference in creating secure relationships. Therefore, it is critically important that we learn to make and receive repair attempts in order to repair the damage that these ruptures create. Many researchers[11,13] on couple relationships, as well as parental relationships

---

[a]This distinction between mechanical and complex adaptive systems may become less clear in the emerging world of artificial intelligence.

with children, have found that the capacity to reach out with sincere remorse or an apology for the injury, while extremely important, is not as critical as the acceptance of that bid for reconciliation on the part of the one who was hurt. Making and, in particular, accepting a repair attempt is perhaps the most important set of skills that we can learn to form the secure foundation necessary for creating nurturing and loving relationships. It is worth noting that the request for a repair must come from a sincere desire to connect with and understand the perspective of the one who felt hurt or injured in some way. It does not work if the repair request is superficial or not perceived as coming from a place of curiosity for what happened and a deep remorse for the hurt, with an intention to learn and do it differently in the future.

Relationships with children

We would like to note that the principles we have described in this article apply to relationships throughout the life span. Children, in particular, are vulnerable to experiences in which they do not feel a sense of safety and security. Like all of us, they yearn to be seen, heard, understood, and valued, leading to a feeling that they are a source of delight for their parents. When parents are overwhelmed by their own needs and stressors, they may find themselves turning away (manifested as wanting their children to manage their own needs without being bothered to interact with them) or turning against (manifested by irritation and annoyance at the needs of their children). Thankfully, like all of us, it is the capacity to repair these moments of misalignment that allow children to reclaim and restore a sense of security with their parents.

SUMMARY

The information provided in this brief article is intended to be an invitation to learn more. The science of Interpersonal Neurobiology (the science of relationships) has expanded and evolved over the past decade, and we have more information available to us now than ever to help us learn better ways of partnering and thriving in our relationships. And importantly, these same skills can be applied to our work teams with resounding success. Readers who are interested in learning more can likely find many good books and articles on the science of relationships. In addition, it is valuable to consult a relationship coach, and there are now an increasing number of coaches who also understand the context of a profession in cardiothoracic surgery.

DISCLOSURE

None of the authors have any relevant disclosures.

REFERENCES

1. Bremner RM, Ungerleider RM, Ungerleider J, et al. Well-being of Cardiothoracic Surgeons in the Time of COVID-19: A Survey by the Wellness Committee of the American Association of Thoracic Surgery. Semin Thorac Cardiovasc Surg 2022;14:S1043.
2. Ungerleider JD, Ungerleider RM, James L, et al. Assessment of the well-being of significant others of cardiothoracic surgeons. J Thorac Cardiovasc Surg 2023;7:396–402.
3. Waldinger R, Schulz M. The good life: lessons from the world's longest scientific study of happiness. New York: Simon and Schuster; 2023.
4. Coan JA, Schaefer HS, Davidson RJ. Lending a Hand: Social Regulation of the Neural Response to Threat. Psychol Sci 2006;17(12):1032–9.
5. Cassidy J. The Nature of the Child's Ties. In: Cassidy J, Shaver P, editors. Handbook of attachment: theory, research, and clinical applications. New York: Guilford Press; 2016. p. 3–39.
6. Siegel D. The developing mind: how relationships and the brain interact to shape who we are. New York: Guilford Press; 1999.
7. Ungerleider RM, Ungerleider JD, Strand A. Discovering Your Mindful Heart: an Explorer's Guide. Developing your internal resources to manage life's demands. Indianapolis: Balboa Press; 2020.
8. Siegel DJ, Bryson TP. The Power of Showing Up: How Parental Presence Shapes Who Our Kids Become and How Their Brains Get, Wired. New York: Ballantine Books; 2021.
9. Beckes L, Coan JA. Social Baseline Theory: The Role of Social Proximity in Emotion and Economy of Action. Social and Personality Psychology Compass 2011;5(12):976–88.
10. Ham J, Tronick E. Infant Resilience to the Stress of the Still-Face. Ann N Y Acad Sci 2006;1094(1):297–302.
11. Gottman J, Silver N. The seven principles for making marriage work. New York: Three Rivers Press; 1999.
12. Gottman J. The science of trust. New York: W.W. Norton; 2011.
13. Wile DB. After the fight: using your disagreements to build a stronger relationship. New York: Guilford Press; 1993.
14. Wile DB. Collaborative Couple Therapy. In: Gurman AS, Jacobson NS, editors. Clinical handbook of couple therapy. New York: Guilford Press; 2002. p. 281–307.
15. Tatkin S. Wired For Love: How understanding your partner's brain and attachment style can help you defuse conflict and build a securee relationship. Oakland, CA: New Harbinger Publications, Inc; 2011.

16. Harms PD. Adult Attachment Styles in the Workplace. Hum Resour Manag Rev 2011;21:285–96.

17. Siegel D. IntraConnected: MWe (me + we): as the integration of self, identity, and belonging. New York: W. W. Norton; 2023.

18. Siegel DJ. Mindsight. New York: Random House Bantam Books; 2010.

19. Dweck CS. Mindset: the new psychology of success. New York: Bantam Books; 2008.

20. Schulz K. Being wrong: adventures in the margin of error. New York: Harper Collins; 2010.

21. Mcraney D, How Minds Change. The surprising science of belief, opinion and persuasion. New York: Portfolio/Penguin; 2022.

22. Edmondson AC. The fearless organization: creating psychological safety in the workplace for learning, innovation and growth. Hoboken, New Jersey: John Wiley & Sons; 2019.

23. Clark TR. The 4 stages of psychological safety. Oakland, CA: Berrett-Koehler Publishers, Inc.; 2020.

24. Gottman J.M. and Making Relationships Work, Harvard Business Review, 2007, 45–50.

25. Siegel DJ. Pocket guide to interpersonal neurobiology: an integrative handbook of the mind. New York: W. W. Norton & Co; 2012.

26. Marcus LJ, Mcnulty EJ, Henderson JM, et al. You're it. Crisis, change, and how to lead when it matters most. , New York: Public Affairs; 2019.

Well-being Through the Synergy of Community Engagement, Health Equity, and Advocacy

Hollis Hutchings, MD[a], Parnia Behinaein, MS[b,1], Ikenna Okereke, MD[c,*]

KEYWORDS

- Community engagement • Mentorship • Equity • Diversity • Health advocacy
- Cardiothoracic surgery

KEY POINTS

- The mentorship of students during the infancy of their education, particularly those from marginalized racial and gender groups, is imperative to promoting diversity.
- A diverse health care workforce confers multifaceted benefits. It reflects the heterogeneous backgrounds of patients and enhances health care professionals' capacity for empathy.
- Caregivers with diverse backgrounds can help mitigate these discrepancies, improving health outcomes for patients of all backgrounds.
- Nonprofit organizations have a role in advancing equity and community engagement. The partnership between the Okereke Foundation, the Department of Surgery, and Henry Ford exemplifies how nonprofits can collaborate.
- Numerous nonprofit organizations nationwide are aligning with surgical departments to champion health equity, diversity in health care, and creative ways to achieve these goals.

INTRODUCTION

Well-being is a quality of positive physical, mental, and social experiences. Well-being allows realization of optimal work and life potential. For cardiothoracic surgeons, core principles of well-being include interconnectivity (fostering relationships), social relatedness to the work we do (service to build a community), and safety (creating a culture for everyone to thrive). Unfortunately, the health care industry suffers from significant racial and gender disparities that negatively affect overall patient care. These disparities persist and have worsened in some aspects. The lack of representation of certain populations in medicine is a result of decades of inequities, broad discrimination, and poor access to equal educational and professional opportunities. To combat these disparities, individuals within medicine and medical institutions should act as advocates for underrepresented communities. We highlight current and future programs that can serve as blueprints to improve health equity, diversity in medicine, and well-being among individuals, health organizations, and communities.

[a] Henry Ford Health, 2799 West Grand Boulevard, Detroit, MI 48202, USA; [b] School of Medicine, Wayne State University, 540 Canfield Street, Detroit, MI 48201, USA; [c] Department of Surgery, Thoracic Surgery, Henry Ford Health, 2799 West Grand Boulevard, Detroit, MI 48202, USA
[1] Present address: 2799 West Grand Boulevard, Detroit, MI 48202.
* Corresponding author.
E-mail address: iokerek1@hfhs.org

Thorac Surg Clin 34 (2024) 281–290
https://doi.org/10.1016/j.thorsurg.2024.04.005

HISTORY
Racial and Gender Biases at the Community Level

Systemic racism is a pervasive force throughout communities, hometowns, workplaces, and social settings. Fellow citizens have assumptions forced on them purely because of external biases not inherent to personal identity. One sees these prejudices highlighted in many ways at the community level. In the not-too-distant past, "Jim Crow laws," or racial segregation laws, were used by local governments to control the presence of African Americans. These laws were designed to prevent African Americans from access to businesses, voting, home loans, and other benefits. Jim Crow laws bled into the coverage provided for veterans and their families under the GI Bill, which was created to provide financial and educational benefits to returning World War II veterans. The distribution of funds was flawed, however, and preferentially were steered away from African Americans. The law failed to provide the same benefits experienced by White veterans to African American veterans, and thus led to this bill being described by some as "affirmative action for Whites."[1,2] Although the Civil Rights Act of 1964 prohibited some of these laws, there are still lingering effects of segregation that are felt today and affect representation in medicine. The housing and school segregation resulting from the Jim Crow laws has created significant inequities in educational opportunities based on race. These inequities persist in today's society and can cause educational deficiencies in African American children early in life.

Redlining was one of the most impactful means of achieving segregation in urban communities. Redlining was a discriminatory policy by the Federal Housing Administration of dividing metropolitan areas into different zones from A to D. Zone A was considered the most desirable and were generally comprised of White Americans. Zone D, alternatively, consisted of the least desirable parts of the community and was reserved for African Americans. These Zone D areas tended to be in the older parts and center of the city. Banks would often deny loans to African American residents of Zone D while granting loans to White Americans in other zones, even if their incomes were equal. Reverse-redlining occurred when the same loans provided to higher income communities were provided to African Americans at inflated rates, again because of perceived hazardous investment climate in African American communities. The infiltration of systemic racism has spurred long-lasting inequities experienced by members of these communities. These practices have led to a consistent lack of resources in African American communities and exacerbated such conditions as food insecurity, poor housing conditions, and lack of high-speed Internet.

Lower income neighborhoods are often subjected to lower quality school systems. Because property taxes are less, surrounding educational facilities receive less funding than other higher income communities.[3] According to the nonprofit group Share Our Strength, directors of the No Kid Hungry initiative, nearly 60% of children from low-income communities reported they had come to school hungry.[4] Hunger in students negatively impacts their ability to focus on school, negatively impacts academic performance, increases behavior problems, and is significantly correlated with childhood illness.[5]

Disparities in the Criminal Justice System

Citizens of racial and ethnic minority groups are often treated differently by the US criminal justice system. This has been highlighted by several monumental cases in the last 10 years, including George Floyd, Breonna Taylor, Ta'Kiya Young and her unborn child, and the thousands of other African American victims of police brutality. African Americans are more likely to be stopped for traffic violations, more likely to be shot by police, and more likely to experience police brutality than White Americans.[6] Geier and colleagues[7] conducted a study of traumatically injured African Americans presenting to a Level 1 trauma center and the impact of discrimination by police on recovery from injury. The authors observed that patients who reported more frequent discrimination demonstrated lower emotional and physical well-being 6 months after injury. Additionally, these same patients reported more severe symptoms of posttraumatic stress disorder 6 months after injury. African American citizens face incarceration at five to seven times higher rates for nonviolent offenses, such as drug possession or selling, more frequently than White citizens.[8] Additionally, African Americans accounted for more than half of inmates facing yearlong or greater sentences for drug-related offenses.[8] The persistent racial biases that plague the legal system introduce the idea that racial majority groups are good, intelligent, and well to do, whereas members of racial minority groups are to be thought of as criminals, in need of rehabilitation, and deserving of punishment.

Childhood and Secondary Education

Disparities in medicine start well before entry into the health care system. Minority children are often at a disadvantage from their majority peers, and these obstacles make acceptance into medical school and obtaining jobs with high-earning potential difficult. In a study by Morgan and colleagues,[9] a longitudinal cohort of 7757 racially diverse children was followed to understand the differences in educational competency. The authors observed large gaps in general knowledge evident at the kindergarten level for African American and Hispanic children compared with their White and Asian counterparts. Additionally, kindergarten general knowledge was the strongest predictor of first grade general knowledge, which in turn was the strongest predictor of a child's science achievement measures in third through eighth grades. Predictors of these disparities included sociodemographic factors; parent attentiveness; the racial, ethnic, and economic composition of the school; and school academic climate. Racial minority children also face stronger punishments for minor infractions, leading to unnecessary absences from school and negative impacts on their education. Del Toro and Wang[10] analyzed 2381 students in sixth, eighth, and tenth grade. This study observed that 26% of minority students with minor infractions (eg, cell phone use, dress code violations) were punished with suspension as opposed to 2% of nonminority students committing the same infractions. The loss of time in school affects students' ability to maintain a pace of learning with their peers. The time away from school affects performance in school level and national level testing and limits future possibilities for higher education. Moreover, the inequity of differential treatment creates mistrust in the education system and may negatively impact students' willingness to pursue fields that demand higher education including master's and doctorate degrees, continuing the racial and ethnic disparities currently experienced in health care. In higher education, the racial disparities persist with only 7% of Ivy League undergraduate students identifying as African American.[11]

Medical Education

The disparities experienced in childhood education continue into medical education and residency positions. Strikingly, we have experienced worsened racial disparities from the 1900s to now. A recent study examined diversity of the National Medical Student Body and showed that the African American male percentage of medical students from 1978 to 2019 dropped from 3.1% to 2.9%.[12] This disappointing statistic illustrates that despite efforts to reduce racial disparities among health care providers, there is still much work to be done. Moreover, gender disparities in medical

education are equally concerning and warrant serious attention. Women face unique challenges that impact their journey through medical education and into professional practice.[13] This is evidenced by the lower enrollment of women in certain medical specialties and the persistent gender pay gap in medicine. Research shows that female medical students and residents often encounter gender bias, which can manifest as unequal opportunities for mentorship, sponsorship, and career advancement.[14] Additionally, there is a notable underrepresentation of women in leadership roles within medical institutions, which further perpetuates these disparities.[15] Addressing these gender-based disparities is crucial for creating a more equitable and inclusive medical community. These disparities continue into postgraduate training among general surgery and cardiothoracic surgery residents. When looking at matched residents, there is a discrepancy in the percentage of applicants of different racial and ethnic groups to the percentage of matched applicants. A poll of 9276 surgery residents was conducted and demonstrated geographic differences in diversity of residents in general surgery programs.[16] Female residents ranged from 38% to 46% depending on region, and Hispanic residents ranged from 7.3% to 8.3%. For residents entering integrated cardiothoracic training programs, there has been no significant change in percentage of African American trainees in the last 15 years. Since the inception of the integrated cardiothoracic pathway, only 2.2% of trainees have been African American.[17] In addition to biases faced when applying for positions, we see these racial and gender biases persist into training positions. A recent systematic review was conducted to understand the presence of gender and racial biases in surgical resident evaluations. In this review, 53 studies met inclusion criteria.[18] In most studies included in their review, disadvantages existed for female trainees regarding standardized examinations, self-evaluations, and program evaluations. Four of the studies assessed racial bias, and all of them observed disadvantages for underrepresented racial minorities who were surgical trainees. In the training of surgical residents, there are also racial disparities in the number of surgical cases that a trainee performs during their residency. A recent study demonstrated that in a racially diverse cohort of 1343 residents, African American residents performed an average of 76 fewer total cases and 69 fewer surgeon junior cases than White residents.[19] Although each racial group performed more cases throughout the 10-year study period, the increase per year remained less for African American residents than for White residents.

Disparities in Academia

Promotion of physicians in academia is an important step toward heightened research opportunities, influence in departments, and opportunities for leadership at a higher level. The first African American female department chair in an academic surgical institution was not until 2021 when KMarie King was appointed Chair of Surgery at Albany Medical Center. She was followed by Andrea Hayes who was appointed Chair of Surgery at Howard University, a historically Black college and university.[20] In a study conducted from 2003 to 2006, most assistant and associate professors of surgery were White (62% and 75%, respectively). African American assistant professors of surgery had lower 10-year promotion rates, and retention rates were lower for minority faculty as compared with their White colleagues.[21] This trend was again seen in a study using American Association of Medical Colleges faculty rosters of US allopathic medical schools. African American and Hispanic faculty were underrepresented in most specialties and were more underrepresented in 2016 than 1990 across all ranks of professorship except for African American females in obstetrics and gynecology. White females were also more underrepresented in many specialties with some subspecialties, with a temporal trend toward worsened disparities.[22]

DEFINITIONS

To develop effective solutions for disparities in medicine, it is important to understand the true level of the dilemma. Next are some examples of the low rates of representation in health care.

1. Cardiothoracic surgeon demographics[23]
   o Race
     ▪ White: 76.6%
     ▪ Asian: 12.7%
     ▪ Hispanic or Latino: 5.0%
     ▪ Black or African American: 1.8%
     ▪ Unknown: 3.8%
   o Gender
     Male: 58.1%
     Female: 41.9%
2. Disparities in treatment patterns
   o Esophageal cancer: African Americans, along with other minority groups, are more likely to be diagnosed at advanced stages of esophageal cancer compared with Whites. Across all stages, minority groups, including African Americans, are less likely to receive surgery for esophageal cancer. Despite this, Hispanics and Asians tend to have improved survival compared with Whites, whereas African Americans experience the worst overall survival.[24]
     ▪ Lung cancer screening: National guidelines for lung cancer screening based on age and smoking exposure are less effective for African Americans compared with White populations. This is attributed to African Americans typically developing lung cancers at a younger age and after less smoking exposure. Only about 32% of African Americans with lung cancer were eligible for screening under the 2013 guidelines, compared with 56% of White individuals. After the 2021 revisions to the guidelines, the eligibility-to-incidence ratio for lung cancer screening was significantly lower for African Americans (9.5) compared with White individuals (20.3).[25]
3. Enrollment in clinical trials
   o There has been a historical lack of diversity in early phase clinical trial accrual, including insufficient representation of racial minorities and women. From 2000 to 2022, the proportion of minority patients in National Cancer Institute-sponsored early phase clinical trials increased only slightly. As an example, the proportion of non-Hispanic Black participants increased from 6.3% to 7.1%.[26,27]

SOLUTIONS AND ADVOCACY
Pipeline Programs

A common criticism from those who are interested in reducing disparities is that there are not enough qualified applicants, as a result of many of the factors described previously. Pipeline programs are designed to increase the number of underrepresented people who have been given the training required to succeed in surgical disciplines. Because the educational disparities and "leaky pipeline" phenomenon begin early in life, these pipeline programs should be targeted toward younger students. Surgical departments and divisions are ideal in many ways to conduct these programs. Because much of surgery has transitioned to minimally invasive approaches, surgeons have the ability to show students surgical techniques and cases on monitors with high definition. Younger generations, who are more inclined to be visual learners, tend to respond favorably to this type of education. In addition, most surgical departments have simulation centers that allow for hands-on activities for students. Our institution has conducted a high school mentorship program for the last 8 academic years.[28] The mentorship program consists of three phases. In phase I, surgeons from our program go to local high schools and discuss life as a surgeon, requirements to become a surgeon, pitfalls and obstacles, potential discrimination faced, and other details. In phase II, high school students attend our simulation center and participate in simulation activities. Simulation activities include peg transfer, robotic ring rollercoaster, and suturing skills. In phase III, selected students are awarded a summer internship. They are paired with an attending surgeon mentor and attend operating room cases and outpatient clinic. The students are paid a stipend of $1000 during the summer. Students who have participated in the program have reported an increased level of self-confidence, a desire to become a surgeon, and an increased belief that they have the dexterity necessary to succeed in surgery. At the end of the program, students submit a summative essay describing their experiences. A graphical representation of word frequency showed that the words "opportunity" and "experience" were among the most used words by the students (**Fig. 1**).

In addressing the challenge of underrepresentation in medicine and promoting diversity within the surgical field, several other notable programs have been created with unique foci and approaches (**Table 1**). The Carlos A. Pellegrini Diversity Visiting Student Internships Program at the University of Washington targets students from diverse backgrounds, offering hands-on experience with surgical teams at renowned medical centers.[29] This initiative exemplifies the impact of early exposure to health care careers, broadening students' perspectives on various medical specialties. Similarly, the Clinical Anatomy Summer Program at Stanford University provides high school students with a comprehensive introduction to a range of medical fields.[30] This program underscores the importance of early education in health care. The University of Alabama at Birmingham's Department of Surgery focuses on research experiences, underscoring the importance of early scientific

inquiry and health care research while offering a foundational understanding of the medical sciences research process.[31] Johns Hopkins Medicine's Surgery Apprenticeship Program sets a precedent for high school programs by focusing on early surgical experiences and research, serving as a valuable model for future initiatives.[32] University of California Irvine Health's Department of Urology offers a Summer Surgery Program that provides hands-on learning opportunities with advanced surgical technologies, inspiring the next generation of medical professionals.[33] The Surgery Clinical Research Continuum at the University of Wisconsin-Madison, supported by the Doris Duke Charitable Foundation and the Department of Surgery, offers a unique pathway that emphasizes clinical research in surgery for high school to college students.[34] Tufts University's Mini Med School engages high school students through hands-on activities, medical simulation exercises, and trips to medical campuses. Their program focuses on medicine, research, and science, thus fostering early interest in these fields.[35] The University of Washington's Neurologic Surgery Summer Student Program, offering an 8-week program with stipends and housing, provides high school students interested in neurologic surgery with an immersive experience.[36] Stanford Medicine's StaRS program, a 7-week summer internship in plastic and reconstructive surgery, caters to high school and undergraduate students, expanding their understanding of this specialized field.[37] Lastly, the Rady Children's Hospital-San Diego Summer Medical Academy, a 2-week program for high school students, provides practical experience and learning in key medical topics, furthering their interest in medical training and practice.[38] Although this list is not comprehensive, each of these programs represents a crucial step toward diversifying the field of surgery. They collectively demonstrate the impact of early educational interventions in

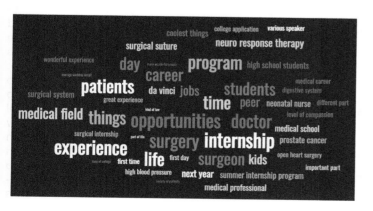

Fig. 1. Word cloud of summative essays from phase III summer interns.

Table 1
Overview of nationwide high school mentorship and engagement programs in surgical departments

Program Name	Institution	Description
Henry Ford Health Department of Surgery High School Mentorship Program	Henry Ford Health	Open to Detroit-area high school students interested in a career in medicine, this program runs during the academic year and offers a $1000 paid summer internship to 10 selected students.
Carlos A. Pellegrini Diversity Visiting Student Internships Program	University of Washington	A funded program for students from diverse backgrounds. Offers a 4-week experience with surgical teams at Seattle Children's Hospital or the University of Washington Medical Center, focusing on diversity in surgery.
Clinical Anatomy Summer Program	Stanford University	Aimed at high school students interested in medical and health-related fields, covering medicine, surgery, dentistry, and other health professions. A comprehensive approach to early medical education.
Summer Research Programs	University of Alabama at Birmingham Department of Surgery	Summer research programs for high school and undergraduate students, such as the Pre-College Research Internship for Students from Minority Backgrounds and the Surgery Undergraduate Research Experience, focusing on hands-on health care research.
Surgery Apprenticeship Program	Johns Hopkins Medicine	Although primarily for undergraduates, this program emphasizes early surgical experiences and research, serving as a model for high school initiatives.
Summer Surgery Program	UC Irvine Health - Department of Urology	Offers exposure to advanced surgical technologies and operating room protocols, providing a unique learning opportunity for aspiring medical professionals.
High C. Surgery Clinical Research Continuum	University of Wisconsin-Madison	Supported by the Doris Duke Charitable Foundation and the University of Wisconsin Department of Surgery, this program offers a unique pathway for high school to college students, emphasizing clinical research in surgery.
Mini Med School	Tufts University	Engages high school students through hands-on activities, medical simulation exercises, and trips to medical campuses, focusing on medicine, research, and science, thus fostering early interest in these fields.
Neurologic Surgery Summer	University of Washington	An 8-wk program with stipends and housing, providing high school students interested in neurologic surgery with an immersive experience.

(continued on next page)

Table 1
(continued)

Program Name	Institution	Description
STaRS Internship Program	Stanford Medicine	A 7-wk summer internship in plastic and reconstructive surgery, catering to high school and undergraduate students, expanding their understanding of this specialized field.
Medical Academy	Rady Children's Hospital	A 2-wk program for high school students at Rady Children's Hospital-San Diego, offering practical experience and learning in key medical topics, furthering their interest in medical training and practice.

inspiring and preparing the next generation of medical professionals.

Institutional Strategies

Surgical departments should consider assigning relative value units to efforts to reduce disparities and improve diversity. Currently, most surgeons who conduct these efforts do so without compensation and alongside their other responsibilities, including clinical relative value unit targets and research productivity requirements. Diversity and equity programs should also be considered a "pillar" when considering academic promotion from assistant professor to associate professor and full professor. This would not only recognize the vital role these programs play in shaping the future of surgery but also incentivize more surgeons to participate in and lead such initiatives.[39]

Multi-Institutional Collaborations

Multi-institutional collaborations are another critical avenue for expanding the impact of diversity and equity initiatives. By partnering with other institutions, departments of surgery can share best practices and enhance the effectiveness of their programs. These collaborations can take various forms, such as joint mentorship programs, shared research projects focusing on diversity in surgery, and combined efforts in advocacy and policy-making. Such collaborative efforts not only provide a broader platform for these important initiatives but also facilitate the pooling of data and experiences, leading to more robust research and more informed policy decisions. By working together, institutions can more effectively address the systemic issues that contribute to disparities in surgery and health care at large, ultimately leading to a more diverse, equitable, and inclusive surgical community.[40]

DISCUSSION

We strongly believe that equitable health care is within reach. Achieving this equity requires a sustained effort from multiple fronts to achieve fairness in treatment. As we strive for improved diversity and inclusion, we have to understand and be mindful of different cultural beliefs within medical facilities. In cardiothoracic surgery, we have previously identified the continued lack of racial diversity in trainees and difficulties for underrepresented minorities in cardiothoracic surgery to advance academically in their postgraduate careers. The first step to addressing this problem in cardiothoracic surgery is emphasizing the truth behind the disparities. At the 2023 American Association for Thoracic Surgery Annual Meeting, one of the podium sessions titled "Bridging the Gap in CT Surgery" focused specifically on diversity and inclusion. This session was well attended and included presentations on gender and racial differences in cardiothoracic surgery. For a larger impact in cardiothoracic surgery, we urge the scientific chairs or committees of large international conferences to select original research presentations focused on diversity and inclusion for presidential sessions and keynote addresses. By reaching a larger audience, we can help elevate the discussion of gender and racial equity within cardiothoracic surgery. Additionally, we urge department chairs and residency/fellowship program directors to invest time in learning the current level of gender and racial disparities in cardiothoracic trainees. There are qualified applicants from all races, genders, and backgrounds applying for fellowship positions, supported by evidence presented in this review. By heightening the awareness of those in positions of power to accept candidates, a more just evaluation of applicants may be accomplished. Finally, the implementation of pipeline programs like the one modeled at our institution can elevate young learners who may not have realized their potential to consider fields in medicine and cardiothoracic surgery. It is easier to visualize one's future when able to draw on a person who shares the same gender or racial background. A common motto applicable to this role-modeling approach is "if you can see it, you can be it." By demonstrating to children, high schoolers, collegiate, and medical students that there are cardiothoracic surgeons who share parts of their background, we may elevate these students to pursue careers in cardiothoracic surgery.

A multilevel approach to patient care may address the disparities currently experienced by members of racial minority groups, notably African American patients. Evidence has demonstrated that African American patients experience later diagnoses of lung cancers and diagnoses at more advanced stages. African Americans also are less likely to receive surgery stage for stage and have worse overall survival compared with White patients. We recommend a tiered approach to reduce the disparities experienced by African American patients. Community engagement is paramount, because acceptance from community partners has been demonstrated to elevate patient awareness of disease and willingness to participate in lung cancer screening and other entry-level interventions. Our group has found success with intervening at the community church level through implementation of interactive kiosks, and direct engagement between members of the health care community and parishioners.[41] Community engagement allows for the development of trust between medical providers and patients and can act as the first step toward seeking treatment. In addition to community engagement, advocacy at the local government level by health care providers and local stakeholders can further access to equitable care.[42] By approaching local government officials and appealing to state and national representatives, funding for city and county level interventions may be obtained, further providing avenues to increase health equity among minority groups. Finally, we recommend exploring a community liaison to function as a bridge between medical centers and at-risk community residents. This liaison may be a nurse, social worker, or other allied health professional who can specifically target neighborhoods and/or patients who have poor access to health care institutions. Through epidemiologic research, we can identify regions in which residents tend not to seek regular medical care and regions with disproportionately higher smoking rates or environmental exposures. Within these regions, community liaisons can intervene directly by providing education, opportunities for screening, and additional assistance.

Advancement of research in cardiothoracic fields should include all patient populations. Historically, African American patients have been hesitant to participate in scientific research trials. The continued mistrust from the Tuskegee Syphilis Study and other research studies that mistreated African Americans has tarnished the relationship between scientific research and the racial minority community.[43] We need to be proactive in rebuilding this broken relationship to serve a diverse group of patients more effectively. The National Lung Screening Trial included only 4.4% of participants as African American, even though African Americans compose 12.6% of the US population.

SUMMARY

We currently practice in a system with health inequity and disparate opportunities for people to enter the health care workforce. These disparities are related to decades of systemic discrimination at the federal, state, and local levels. Through creative, community-based programs, cardiothoracic surgeons can have a meaningful impact on the health and opportunity of people with the greatest need. We have demonstrated how influencing the lives of underrepresented youth can create a pipeline of skilled personnel in health care and a diverse workforce poised to combat inequities in health care delivery. Furthermore, collaboration among institutions committed to health equity will lead to dissemination of valuable interventions that can improve the health of more people. By striving for health equity and workforce diversity, cardiothoracic surgeons can add value to the work we do, create a safe environment for people to thrive and create interconnectivity with our communities, thus enhancing our own well-being.

DISCLOSURE

The authors have nothing to disclose.

REFERENCES

1. Katznelson I. Poverty and race. Pov Race Act Coun 2006;15:1–5.
2. Policy H. When affirmative action was white. History & Policy. 2005. Available at: https://www.historyandpolicy.org/policy-papers/papers/when-affirmative-action-was-white. [Accessed 20 November 2023].
3. Galster G, Godfrey E. By words and deeds: racial steering by real estate agents in the U.S. in 2000. J Am Plann Assoc 2005;71(3):251–68.
4. How does hunger affect learning? No Kid Hungry. 2023. Available at: https://www.nokidhungry.org/blog/how-does-hunger-affect-learning#:~:text=In%

20a%20preeffects%20of%20hunger%20as%20well. [Accessed 22 November 2023].

5. Kleinman RE, Hall S, Green H, et al. Diet breakfast and academic performance in children. Ann Nutr Metab 2002;46(Suppl 1):24–30.

6. Schwartz SA. Police brutality and racism in America. Explore 2020;16(5):280–2.

7. Geier TJ, Timmer-Murillo SC, Brandolino AM, et al. History of Racial Discrimination by Police Contributes to Worse Physical and Emotional Quality of Life in Black Americans After Traumatic Injury. J Racial Ethn Health Disparities 2023;1–9. https://doi.org/10.1007/s40615-023-01649-8.

8. Carson E. A. & Sabol W. J. (2012). Prisoners in 2011. NCJ 239808(11) 1

9. Morgan PL, Farkas G, Hillemeier MM, et al. Science achievement gaps begin very early persist and are largely explained by modifiable factors. Educ Res 2016;45(1):18–35.

10. Del Toro Juan, Ming-Te Wang. Vicarious severe school discipline predicts racial disparities among non-disciplined Black and White American adolescents. Child Dev 2023. https://doi.org/10.1111/cdev.13958.

11. Ede-Osifo Uwa. A debate brews among Black Ivy League students over representation on campus. NBC News. 2023. Available at: https://www.nbcnews.com/news/nbcblk/debate-brews-black-ivy-league-students-representation-campus-rcna117726. [Accessed 22 November 2023].

12. Morris DB, Gruppuso PA, McGee HA, et al. Diversity of the national medical student body: four decades of inequities. N Engl J Med 2021;384(17):1661–8.

13. Miller VM, Padilla LA, Swicord WB, et al. Gender differences in cardiothoracic surgery interest among general surgery applicants. Ann Thorac Surg 2021; 112(3):961–7.

14. Winkel AF, Telzak B, Shaw J, et al. The role of gender in careers in medicine: a systematic review and thematic synthesis of qualitative literature. J Gen Intern Med 2021;36(8):2392–9.

15. Bryan DS, Debarros M, Wang SX, et al. Gender trends in cardiothoracic surgery authorship. J Thorac Cardiovasc Surg 2023;166(5):1375–84.

16. Kearse LE, Jensen RM, Schmiederer IS, et al. Diversity equity and inclusion: a current analysis of general surgery residency programs. Am Surg 2022; 88(3):414–8.

17. Powell M, Wilder F, Obafemi O, et al. Trends in diversity in integrated cardiothoracic surgery residencies. Ann Thorac Surg 2022;114(3):1044–8.

18. Helliwell LA, Hyland CJ, Gonte MR, et al. Bias in surgical residency evaluations: a scoping review. J Surg Educ 2023;80(7):922–47.

19. Eruchalu CN, Etheridge JC, Hammaker AC, et al. Racial and Ethnic Disparities in Operative Experience Among General Surgery Residents: A Multi-Institutional Study from the US ROPE Consortium. Ann Surg 2024;279(1):172–9.

20. Bajaj SS, Tu L, Stanford FC. Superhuman but never enough: Black women in medicine. Lancet 2021; 398(10309):1398–9.

21. Abelson, Wong NZ, Symer M, et al. Racial and ethnic disparities in promotion and retention of academic surgeons. Am J Surg 2018 Oct;216(4):678–82.

22. Lett E, Orji WU, Sebro R, et al. Declining racial and ethnic representation in clinical academic medicine: a longitudinal study of 16 US medical specialties. PLoS One 2018;13(11):e0207274. https://doi.org/10.1371/journal.pone.0207274.

23. Cardiothoracic surgeon demographics and statistics [2023]: Number of cardiothoracic surgeons in the US. Zippia.com. 2021. Available at: https://www.zippia.com/cardiothoracic-surgeon-jobs/demographics/. [Accessed 20 November 2023].

24. Okereke IC, Westra J, Tyler D, et al. Disparities in esophageal cancer care based on race: a National Cancer Database analysis. Dis Esophagus 2022; 35(6):doab083.

25. Choi E, Ding VY, Luo SJ, et al. Risk Model-Based Lung Cancer Screening and Racial and Ethnic Disparities in the US. JAMA Oncol 2023;9(12): 1640–8.

26. Adams-Campbell LL, Ahaghotu C, Gaskins M, et al. Enrollment of African Americans onto clinical treatment trials: study design barriers. J Clin Oncol 2004;22(4):730–4.

27. NCI-sponsored Cancer Clinical Trials Have Become More Diverse Over Past Two Decades. American Association for Cancer Research (AACR). 2023. Available at: https://www.aacr.org/about-the-aacr/newsroom/news-releases/nci-sponsored-cancer-clinical-trials-have-become-more-diverse-over-past-two-decades/. [Accessed 20 November 2023].

28. Hutchings H, Chang D, Ruffin W, et al. Effect of cardiothoracic surgery mentorship on underrepresented high school students. J Thorac Cardiovasc Surg 2024;167(5):1885–90.

29. Department of Surgery. Carlos A. Pellegrini Diversity Visiting Student Internships Program - Department of Surgery. Department of Surgery. 2023. Available at: https://uwsurgery.org/introduction-to-surgical-education3/educationintroduction/div-edu-opps/#:~:text=The%20Diversity%20Visiting%20Student%20Internships,University%20of%20Washington%20Medical. [Accessed 20 November 2023].

30. High School Summer Programs. Surgery. 2023. Available at: https://surgery.stanford.edu/education/Summer-Programs.html. [Accessed 20 November 2023].

31. High Schoolers and Undergraduates - Surgery. Uab.edu. 2023. Available at: https://bb.uab.edu/medicine/surgery/education/high-schoolers-and-undergraduates. [Accessed 20 November 2023].

32. Educational Programs. Hopkinsmedicine.org. 2023. Available at: https://www.hopkinsmedicine.org/surgery/education/#:~:text=,SAP%20Description. [Accessed 20 November 2023].

33. Summer Surgery Program | UC Irvine Health | Department of Urology. Uci.edu. 2020. Available at: https://www.urology.uci.edu/education_summersurgery.shtml. [Accessed 20 November 2023].

34. High C. Surgery Clinical Research Continuum: High School to College Program - Department of Surgery. Department of Surgery. 2023. Available at: https://www.surgery.wisc.edu/education-training/training-for-researchers/surgery-clinical-research-continuum-high-school-to-college-program/. [Accessed 21 November 2023].

35. Mini Med School. University College. 2023. Available at: https://universitycollege.tufts.edu/high-school/programs/mini-med-school-choice. [Accessed 21 November 2023].

36. Neurological Surgery Summer Student Program | UW Department of Neurological Surgery. Uw.edu. 2023. Available at: https://neurosurgery.uw.edu/education/summer-student-programs. [Accessed 21 November 2023].

37. STaRS Internship Program. Division of Plastic & Reconstructive Surgery. 2022. Available at: https://plasticsurgery.stanford.edu/research/stars.html. [Accessed 21 November 2023].

38. Medical Academy | Rady Children's Hospital. Rchsd.org. 2023. Available at: https://www.rchsd.org/programs-services/center-for-healthier-communities/youth-development/medical-academy/. [Accessed 21 November 2023].

39. Childers CP, Dworsky JQ, Russell MM, et al. Association of work measures and specialty with assigned work relative value units among surgeons. JAMA Surg 2019;154(10):915–21.

40. West MA, Hwang S, Maier RV, et al. Ensuring equity, diversity, and inclusion in academic surgery: an American Surgical Association white paper. Ann Surg 2018;268(3):403–7.

41. Dulchavsky SA, Ruffin WJ, Johnson DA, et al. Use of an interactive, faith-based kiosk by congregants of four predominantly African-American churches in a metropolitan area. Front Public Health 2014;2:106.

42. Mayer J, Murray G. STS advocacy. Ann Thorac Surg 2015;97:S34–9.

43. Scharff DP, Mathews KJ, Jackson P, et al. More than Tuskegee: understanding mistrust about research participation. J Health Care Poor Underserved 2010;21(3):879–97.

Managing Career Transitions in Cardiothoracic Surgery

Dawn S. Hui, MD[a], Jairo Andres Espinosa, MD[b],
Andrea J. Carpenter, MD, PhD[c],*

KEYWORDS

- Career transition • Cardiothoracic surgery • Wellness

KEY POINTS

- At each phase of a surgical career, early preparation for transition to the next is key to success.
- Developing collegial and collaborative relationships should be a focus throughout one's career.
- Retain an understanding of how your personal goals and interests fit into the strategic vision of the department and institution.
- It is crucial to seek legal counsel with expertise in physician employment contracts.
- Preparation for retirement requires early attention and advanced planning of one's financial and personal well-being.

INTRODUCTION

A career in cardiothoracic surgery is a lifelong endeavor of service, dedication, passion, and commitment involving personal growth across multiple domains. While surgical technical skills and judgment are critical to success, so too are skills in building a vision and growth plan in order to achieve personal and professional fulfillment. This article discusses the essential components of managing a career in cardiothoracic surgery, beginning with the critical transition out of practice, through transitions during an established practice, and into retirement.

TRANSITION FROM TRAINING TO PRACTICE

Progressing from trainee to practicing surgeon is one of the most difficult transitions in a surgical career. Early career can be associated with high stress leading to dissatisfaction, job changes, and burnout. Finding the right position for your career goals is critical to success.[1] Most training programs are well designed to prepare the surgeon with knowledge and skill but variable in preparing trainees for the realities of practice.[2] The following guide outlines the basic process to achieve a successful early career. Start the search for the ideal first job at least a year before graduation—the earlier the better. Update your CV and keep it up to date. Seek advice from mentors both internal and external to your training program.

A successful transition to practice begins with an introspective review of personal career and life goals. Identify the aspects of practice experienced during training that you find most satisfying and consider whether you have or want a particular niche in your practice. Decide whether you prefer academic practice, including teaching and research, or a purely clinical practice. Recognize that independent private practices are becoming rare and challenging to navigate immediately after

[a] Department of Cardiothoracic Surgery, Joe R. and Teresa Lozano Long School of Medicine, 7703 Floyd Curl, MC 7841, San Antonio, TX 78229, USA; [b] Southern California Heart Centers, 506 West Valley Boulevard, San Gabriel, CA 91776, USA; [c] Department of Cardiothoracic Surgery, Joe R. and Teresa Lozano Long School of Medicine, MC 7990, San Antonio, TX 78229, USA
* Corresponding author.
E-mail address: carpentera2@uthscsa.edu

Thorac Surg Clin 34 (2024) 291–297
https://doi.org/10.1016/j.thorsurg.2024.04.012
1547-4127/24/© 2024 Elsevier Inc. All rights reserved.

training. Thus, it is most probable that you will start your practicing career as an employed surgeon whether it is in an academic center, multispecialty group, or hospital employment. Include personal and family needs in this review such as an environment amenable to noncareer activities you value, the needs of a growing family, or proximity to your family and support systems. If you are isolated in work and lacking outlets to relieve the stress, you will not be happy.

There are many avenues to identify candidate opportunities. Attend national and regional cardiothoracic meetings to network with fellow surgeons, review "job boards," or attend sessions relevant to your interests. These are good places, along with introductions from faculty in your program, to look for the "hidden job market." Many jobs are not advertised because employers are looking for junior partners relying on word of mouth among their trusted colleagues. Potential opportunities are posted on online resources such as CTSnet, Health eCareers, LinkedIn, or physician recruiting agencies. You may be approached by recruiters about specific opportunities. It is worth your time to talk with them, whether or not the opportunity appeals to you, as they may have others. Health care systems such as Banner Health or HCA list openings on their own Web sites. Academic centers also post jobs on their sites: look for the Human Resources page at institutions where you are interested. Faculty in your training program get job announcements from many sources, including friends and colleagues, so ask them.

When the time comes to interview, go well prepared. They should already have your most recently updated CV, but if you have new items to add be sure to update again and take copies with you. Research the group you will interview with and know about the surgeons, administrators, or other team members you are likely to meet. Get information on the area such as cost of living and activities of interest in the area. Know the expected salary, benefits, and promotion opportunity. Be prepared to ask about call coverage, vacation time, moving expenses, administrative support, start-up funds for research, and support for professional education. Be collegial and respectful, but do not hesitate to talk about the things you value most: asking should not deter the practice where you interview, but failing to ask may lead to later challenges in negotiation. Understand what support and back up you can expect. Remember that you are interviewing them as much as they are interviewing you. After the interview, make notes of the experience and your thoughts for later review.

Learn about physician contracting and have some idea of what is or is not negotiable in each employment environment. For example, an employer may not have discretion regarding institutional policy about vacation for a new hire, or they may be able to negotiate a different benefit that can entice a desired candidate. Once you have an idea of a place or places to consider, meet with an attorney who specializes in physician contracting armed with all the information you have gathered. It is invaluable to enter negotiations prepared with realistic requirements and acceptable choices. Do not sign any letter of intent or contract without reviewing it with counsel. You can easily overlook or dismiss issues that will cause trouble later. Do not rely on oral promises until you see it in writing.

Once you settle on the job and where you will go, plan sometime between residency and your first job. The time is well spent to decompress from the intensity of training and arrive at your new place rested and ready to perform. You will need to bear the cost of interim medical coverage such as COBRA especially if you have children, but starting a new job having recovered from the constant strain of training will pay dividends.

When you start your first job, there are 2 traps to avoid. First, understand that you will need to build a practice by developing the confidence of referring physicians. So do not be surprised if your first few months to a year are not as busy as your last year of training. Second, take care in the selection of cases you tackle. To gain the confidence of referring physicians, you must demonstrate thoughtful decision-making and good surgical results. You likely have not thought about how much your faculty contributed to the success of very complex cases, so do not be shy about asking for help as you build your reputation. Those first complications will feel very personal because they are now yours alone. Get comfortable with your ability, gradually increase the complexity of your work, and you will not fall victim to high stress, dissatisfaction, and early burnout. If you succeeded in the interview stage with understanding the group you are joining, this should not be difficult.

TRANSITIONS DURING CAREER

Once you are established in practice, career transitions can be major opportunities for growth or risks for disruption of growth. In this section, we outline a general framework for transitions that is broadly applicable, whether one is in a purely clinical practice or a surgeon–scientist's practice. A common division of career stages is based on years in practice—early, mid, and late (or senior). These stages correlate to the phases in the "Phase Development Model" of leadership (**Table 1**).[3,4] The rate of personal growth/development and the timing of opportunities for transitions from a formal standpoint (ie, titles or leadership positions) will vary from individual to individual. At the beginning of each stage, one should establish one's developmental priorities and goals, the skillsets on which one wishes to focus, and how these fit into a long-term career plan. This should be done with the guidance of a mentor or mentors. Continual assessment of progress and reassessment of the initial goals and priorities should occur throughout the phase itself. Another framework, described for academic career development, takes a value-based approach by developing 1, 3, and 5 year plans based on your governing values.[5]

Regardless of approach, 4 types of relationships should be evaluated—relationship to self, relationship to peers, relationship to the team, and relationship to the institution. As Gewertz and Logan state, "As physicians move phases, they go through a period of uncertainty" that may require switching of strategies or else risk derailment. A formal departmental program to prepare faculty for professional, personal, and environmental transitions termed "anticipatory guidance" has been described (**Table 2**), with the goal of proactively identifying and rectifying mismatches between individual's skills/interests and job descriptions leading to burnout and inefficiencies.[5] Such an approach requires departmental and institutional commitment. Finally, we discuss considerations in transitions between institutions and physician employment contracts (**Box 1**).

Interinstitutional Transitions: Reasons and Resources

Often, formal career transitions align with institutional changes when opportunities for formal leadership positions open up at another institution or practice. The decision to move from an institution may be tempting during periods of dissatisfaction, leadership change, plateauing of local opportunities, or personal growth. One should carefully and objectively evaluate the reasons for moving and the chances of success. This can be challenging given that the individual cannot fully understand the strategies, culture/values, and local politics of a different institution or practice, or anticipate barriers to success. Extensive research should be undertaken to assess the new institution's strategic plan, whether that plan is attainable and whether it aligns with one's personal goals and values. Also consider the stability of the organization and department, existing leadership, and any planned leadership changes or threats to such. Understand the local market including competing practices and patient populations, opportunities for growth if that is within the mission and within which realms, and the likelihood of attracting successful talent. If multiple entities are involved (such as a hospital system and an academic medical center), gaining understanding or insight into the relationship between the entities and how well their priorities are aligned will be useful for anticipating the power dynamics and challenges to be faced.

Resources for this assessment include discussions with the institution's leadership, current and past personnel, colleagues with similar experiences, mentors, and sponsors. Past personnel may be invaluable in being able to speak with perspective and somewhat more freely about perceived weaknesses or missteps. When to be transparent with one's current employer about interest in or impending plans to leave one's current position is a controversial topic which is outside the scope of this article but one that should be carefully considered. One may request confidentiality from all parties but should never assume that confidentiality will not be violated (whether inadvertently or not).

Table 1
Phase development model of physician leadership

Phase	Description	Priorities	Academic Title
I	Team player	Establishing self and relationships	Assistant professor
II	Team captain	Building a reputation and team	Associate professor
III	Coach	Attracting others	Professor, chair
IV	Team president	Being attracted to new leadership roles	Dean or president
V	Sports commissioner/ league founders	Disrupting others (ie, disruptive change)	Entrepreneur

Adapted from Gewertz, Bruce L.; Logan, Dave C. The Best Medicine: A Physician's Guide to Effective Leadership. Springer New York. Kindle Edition. ISBN 978-1-4939-2219-2.

Table 2
Components of anticipatory guidance faculty development program

Junior Faculty	Mentoring committee of at least 3 members, with one extra-departmental member Short annual report of goals and accomplishments
Midcareer Faculty	One-on-one meetings with division chiefs Formal mentoring committee Leadership development programs
Senior Faculty	Educational sessions on options and strategies to transition roles and percent effort; financial considerations and planning for retirement

Adapted from Schor NF, Guillet R, McAnarney ER. Anticipatory guidance as a principle of faculty development: managing transition and change. Acad Med. 2011;86(10):1235-1240.

Physician Employment Contracts and Negotiations

For most physicians, postresidency will be their first experience with contract negotiations. There will be numerous elements that one has not previously had to consider or negotiate (**Table 3**). The American Medical Association has published guides[6,7] outlining the major areas for consideration. Consultation with legal counsel experienced in physician contracting is well worth the cost to fully understand the complex legal and financial implications of contract terms and to ensure that potential problems or misunderstandings have been identified and, if negotiable, resolved. There is variability among employers in the flexibility of negotiating terms. Agreed upon changes should be confirmed in writing before signing. The negotiating process may reveal red flags such as reneging on terms that were verbally agreed upon terms during the interview process or having unrealistic expectations for call coverage.

Lawyers experienced in physician employment contracts can be found through state medical associations, city or state bar associations, or referrals from other physicians. Specify that you are looking for someone experienced with physician employment contracts. Legal fees and structures vary; be sure to understand the fee structure, rate (hourly vs flat fee), expected number of billable hours, and when the bill is due. Clearly specify what you would like the lawyer to do for you.

Box 1
The phase development model: pearls and pitfalls

Phase I: Early Career

This phase is the beginning of establishing a professional reputation and is critical to setting the trajectory of one's career. In cardiothoracic surgery, it comes at the end of a long period of training, but given the trend toward specialization one should carefully weigh whether the pursuit of additional advanced training will benefit achieving one's goals. Once in clinical practice, the natural focus of an early career surgeon is on his or her individual results and development. This is appropriate, as derailment at this stage can be devastating to one's career. Mentors and partners should be supportive in attaining excellent outcomes, and this should perhaps be the most important consideration of one's first job. However, focus on self should not come at the expense of relationships with others, including peers, support staff, and superiors. Clinical, research, and administrative activity should align with program or department priorities. A reputation not only for clinical excellence but also collegiality is critical to the next phases.

Phase II: Mid-career

The transition to this phase is characterized by a broadening of focus and attitude beyond one's own goals and interests. Success is defined in a way that expands beyond individual results to organizational priorities, and from outcomes themselves (the "what") to the methods and processes that lead to outcomes (the "how"). The individual, having attained local or regional reputation, should transition to mentoring junior partners and eventually attracting talent. Formally evaluating others' performance, managing conflicts, and hiring and firing are new responsibilities. A holistic understanding of the whole team and how individuals' strengths and weaknesses complement each other to attain objectives is key to success. One should be attuned to each individual team member's priorities, motivations, method of operation, and goals. Such tasks should be carried out with the departmental and institutional strategic considerations in mind.

Phase III and Beyond: Late Career

The transition to senior surgeon continues the trend of focusing outward, rather than inward, and expanding your circle of influence and impact. Influence and political capital should be spent to support and empower junior colleagues, peers within other departments that have mutually beneficial goals, and to harbor against or deal with times of crises or threats to resources.

Table 3
Key elements of a physician contract

Obligations	Type and Scope of Medicine Being Practiced Number of hours worked, on-call hours, and availability Expectations and metrics of productivity Clinical and administrative responsibilities
Resources	Operating room availability, support staff, equipment Office space, support staff Marketing, physician liaisons
Compensation structure	Fixed vs variable compensation model Performance benchmarks
Benefits	Health care benefits including dependent policies Retirement benefits including employer contributions Benefits Payment of licensing fees, professional society dues Time off: amount and structure Continuing Medical Education funding Liability and disability insurance: amount and type Medical student loan repayment
Noncompete provisions and restrictive covenants	Duration, proximity, and triggers
Termination	Without vs with cause Advance notice period Reciprocal notice requirement Immediate or automatic termination Patient notice and patient records

Negotiations with the employer can be done by the lawyer or by yourself.

For physicians negotiating a leadership position, the contract should include a commitment from the hospital or institution to provide resources, often termed a "package," that are necessary to the success of the mission. Elements include institutional commitment to support and promote programs, funds and control to hire additional faculty, dedicated operational and administrative staff, access to clinic/laboratory/office space, leadership positions, committee appointments, and other infrastructure or resources needed. An ongoing provision of resources may be contingent on achieving performance metrics specified in the contract, and such metrics should be clearly defined and attainable within a reasonable time frame.

Throughout one's career, one must continuously define and evaluate one's role and relationships within the team, the institution, and the health care system. As your career progresses, you will expand your focus toward broader and broader domains. While a formal job description outlines the scope and expectations associated with your job title, the reality is that there will be many expectations and responsibilities that are unwritten and dictated by the existing culture and power dynamics. This culture, at first, may be foreign to you if you are coming from a different system (especially one with a radically different model and/or culture). Even if you are transitioning within the same system, the complexity of relationships and team dynamics may have been previously undisclosed or unapparent to you. Complicating this is that one is often a member of multiple teams. Identify supportive people, whether they are teammates, mentors, or sponsors, who can help you navigate these challenges.

One should also pay attention to individual differences in leadership and communication styles. When speaking with superiors, it is most effective to tailor your conversations to their agendas and priorities while also clearly making your own priorities and voice are heard. At the same time, reflect on what leadership strengths you possess, what style you wish to develop, and what will be effective for your health care system. Observe and learn from others' experiences. An executive coach may be helpful in planning for and managing career transitions.[8]

TRANSITION TO RETIREMENT

Preparation for retirement should start much earlier during the career than most surgeons consider. Indeed, it is common for a surgeon to arrive at retirement ill-prepared, and absent preparation will delay retirement. Feeling personal identity tied to career, responsibility to patients, financial insecurity, or lack of outside interests is common barriers to retirement.[9,10]

Financial planning is the first key and should begin as soon as the surgeon begins receiving income: "Pay Yourself First" is excellent advice. This requires a 2 pronged approach: dispense debt and save money. Resolving the debt accrued during the years of education and training is generally well understood by newly practicing surgeons. Unfortunately, all that education often does not include an understanding of financial management. Simple savings are not adequate to meet the needs of a long-life in retirement. Begin contributing to retirement plans whether employment-based or individual including individual retirement account, 401(k), 403(b), or pension. Pensions are rare today, but social security is available to all citizens paying taxes. In addition to making contributions, managing the funds effectively is key. For most of us, that requires working with a certified financial advisor and keeping close track of that advisor's performance over time, being prepared to change plans as needed.

The culture of thoracic surgery practice often favors work life over personal and family activities. This culture can foster an unhappy home life, failure to develop noncareer interests, and burnout. Recognize that the duration of a career does not have a defined endpoint, so it is important to modify the approach to work and actively pursue other interests. This includes increasing the time and effort given to pre-existing interests and trying out new activities that contribute to health and wellness.

As stated previously, transition to practice, throughout a career, and to retirement requires defining career goals and metrics that constitute meeting those goals. As your career progresses, these goals may change, new goals may be added, and some goals will be easily met while others prove more elusive. Achieving preplanned goals helps with the decision of when to retire. Recall that a career does not have a predefined endpoint. Meeting goals will help to identify that endpoint. Ideally, we all want to retire while our clinical, technical, and mental capacities are strong, and we can look forward to years of fulfilling retirement. Retiring too early denies the profession a skilled operator and the younger generation the mentorship needed to reach full potential. Retiring too late can be harmful to patients and our health care institutions while also denying ourselves those years of fulfilling life in retirement.

Succession planning is critical to a successful transition to retirement. In fact, failure of succession planning is the most described barrier to retirement in the references listed. Whether succession means transitioning patient care to someone else in a solo practice, negotiating a plan with a specialty or multispecialty group, or assuring that a hospital system or academic practice is prepared for your departure, this is critical. Failed succession may lead to a void if something forces a sudden departure. Ideally, the transition is smoother if there are intermediate steps between a busy full-time career and the beginning of retirement. A good succession plan may take many forms depending on the nature of practice but ideally affords a transition in which senior's talent and experience prepares junior surgeons to move forward seamlessly.

Retirement should not be the end of life's satisfaction. We give up many things to devote time and energy to our careers, and we need to consider what is most important to achieve during retirement. Whether that includes enjoying a happy home life, reveling in the successes of children and grandchildren, traveling the world to experience other cultures and see new sights, or devoting more time to those noncareer activities you have been cultivating it is important to envision what we want in retirement.[11,12]

Plan ahead for where your home will be in retirement. Access to health care as we age is a major aspect in the choice of where to live. The community of family and friends is a critical area to consider whether you choose to live where you worked or seek other places. Before retiring, research cost of living, tax considerations that may impact your retirement income, climate, access to easy travel, and other factors important to you. As you realize meeting your career goals, having plans for the next step will help to define the "when" to retire.

In summary, planning for retirement should encompass an entire career. If you have retired all debt, built a strong financial plan, sustained and grown noncareer interests, defined and met most career goals, and planned a postcareer lifestyle you have the best possible chance to enjoy retirement. The decision of when to retire then can be made with a succession plan in place for your practice and the agreement with the family you acquired along the way. Retirement should just be the beginning of the next adventure in your life.

DISCLOSURE

The authors have nothing to disclose. No funding was provided to supprt this work.

REFERENCES

1. David EA, Nasir BS. Transition to practice, lessons learned: Academic general thoracic surgery. J Thorac Cardiovasc Surg 2016;151(4):920–4. Epub 2015 Dec 19. PMID: 26809422.
2. Sachdeva AK. Educational interventions aimed at the transition from surgical training to surgical practice. Am J Surg 2019;217(3):406–9. Epub 2018 Oct 3. PMID: 30309620.
3. Gewertz BL, Logan DC. The best medicine: a Physician's guide to effective leadership. New York: Springer; 2015.
4. Pololi L. Career development for academic medicine—a nine step strategy. BMJ 2006;332:s38.
5. Schor NF, Guillet R, McAnarney ER. Anticipatory guidance as a principle of faculty development: managing transition and change. Acad Med 2011; 86(10):1235–40.
6. Available at: https://www.ama-assn.org/medical-residents/transition-resident-attending/understanding-physician-employment-contracts. [Accessed 23 January 2024].
7. Available at: https://www.ama-assn.org/medical-residents/transition-resident-attending/physician-contracting-restrictive-covenants. [Accessed 23 January 2024].
8. Hui DS, Rosinia F. The scoop on executive coaching for physicians. blog article for the society of thoracic surgeons. Available at: https://www.sts.org/blog/scoop-executive-coaching-physicians. [Accessed 22 November 2023].
9. Silver MP, Hamilton AD, Biswas A, et al. A systematic review of physician retirement planning. Hum Resour Health 2016;14(1):67. PMID: 27846852; PMCID: PMC5109800.
10. Pannor Silver M, Easty LK. Planning for retirement from medicine: a mixed-methods study. CMAJ Open 2017;5(1):E123–9. PMID: 28401128; PMCID: PMC5378543.
11. Baumgartner WA. The exit strategy: preparing for retirement. Thorac Surg Clin 2024;34(1):105–10. Epub 2023 Sep 15. PMID: 37953047.
12. Rosengart TK, Doherty G, Higgins R, et al. Transition Planning for the Senior Surgeon: Guidance and recommendations from the society of surgical chairs. JAMA Surg 2019;154(7):647–53. Erratum in: JAMA Surg. 2019 Jul 1;154(7):676. PMID: 31090889.

Strategies of Well-being Training and Resilience

Dustin M. Walters, MD[a],*, Michael Maddaus, MD[b]

KEYWORDS

- Resilience • Burnout • Well-being • Wellness • Fulfillment • Belonging

KEY POINTS

- Training ourselves, as surgeons, to be more resilient serves to cope with the challenges we face, but also protects us against burnout.
- Understanding what fulfills us and pursuing fulfilling work activities is fundamental for our happiness.
- Humans have an inherent need for community, connection, and belonging and fostering these has a positive effect on our well-being.
- Mitigation of microstresses and activities that make us feel overwhelmed is important.
- Creating and making frequent deposits into a "resilience bank account" is an important strategy to help us function as our best selves.

INTRODUCTION

It is after 5:00 PM on Friday afternoon and you just finished the last elective case of what has been a long, tiring week. You retreat to the silence of your office and realize everyone else has left for the weekend. What you expected to be a simple 2-hour right upper lobectomy turned into a 5-hour slog of lysis of adhesions due to complete pleural symphysis. The dissection of the pulmonary arteries and lymph nodes was miserable, and you feel exhausted. You know you would feel better if you had slept last night, but you stayed up later than you should have, watching television. And sleep is not the only thing you have neglected as your stomach grumbles, reminding you that you skipped lunch to meet with a student between cases and all you have eaten is a lukewarm cup of weak coffee 10 hours ago. You wryly joke that maybe you will lose a pound or 2, since you have not had the time or energy to exercise, something that you loved but slowly faded into the distance several months ago. You check your phone and realize it is 5:37 PM and your son's basketball game, which you promised him to attend, tipped off 7 minutes ago. You start to dictate the operation and try to multitask by answering emails and encounter 47 unread messages, mostly junk, but a few need attention including the overdue reminder of an assigned manuscript review. Once again, you berate yourself for having agreed to review it in the first place since you *hate* reviewing manuscripts. Two students have emailed reminders about letters of recommendation you still need to write, there are several more messages from colleagues regarding other demands for your time, and your chair wants you to lead some random hospital-level committee, for which you know nothing about and could not care less. You finish dictating and navigate to the electronic medical record (EMR) and are hit by the tsunami of dozens of uncompleted tasks when your phone buzzes with a text from your spouse: "The game just started. What's your estimated time of arrival (ETA)?" A wave of loneliness washes over you, and you feel fried, burned out even. To break the

[a] Department of Surgery, University of Connecticut, 263 Farmington Avenue, MC8073, Farmington, CT 06032, USA; [b] Department of Surgery, University of Minnesota, 2323 West 52nd Street, Minneapolis, MN 55410, USA
* Corresponding author. Department of Surgery, University of Connecticut, 263 Farmington Avenue, Farmington, CT 06030.
E-mail address: dwalters@uchc.edu

Thorac Surg Clin 34 (2024) 299–308
https://doi.org/10.1016/j.thorsurg.2024.04.006
1547-4127/24/© 2024 Elsevier Inc. All rights reserved.

silence and to perk yourself up a bit, you turn on some music. Over the speaker, "Once in a Lifetime" by the Talking Heads drowns out the silence and David Byrne asks, rhetorically, almost too appropriately, "Well, how did I get here?"

The Scope of the Problem

Burnout is common among all physicians and its prevalence has been increasing for decades, peaking during the recent coronavirus disease era.[1] Compared to the average physician, surgeons report similarly high rates of burnout, defined as emotional exhaustion, depersonalization, and decreased effectiveness at work.[2] In a recent study from the American Association for Thoracic Surgery, half of the cardiothoracic surgeons surveyed manifested significant signs of burnout, with 50% reporting a "sense of dread coming to work," high rates of physical (58%) and emotional (50%) exhaustion, and 46% reporting a lack of enthusiasm at their jobs.[3] These numbers are alarming since our core responsibility as surgeons is to show up at work functioning as our best selves so that we can care for those in need.

The problem, however, begins long before we don our attending coats. Studies have shown that medical students and trainees experience similar or increased rates of burnout compared to post-training physicians.[4] Cardiothoracic surgical trainees report high levels of dissatisfaction with balance in their professional lives, with high rates of burnout (>50%), depression, and regret about career choice.[5] The question is why? How do we begin our journeys as intelligent, driven, altruistic people and frequently become shadows of ourselves? And ultimately, what can we do to mitigate this trend? Curbing the burnout epidemic will certainly require a complex, multifaceted approach bringing together individual, health care system, and even national solutions, perhaps even a paradigm shift in the way we deliver health care. A full accounting of these solutions is beyond the scope of this article. Our goal rather, is to offer practical solutions and tools we can employ at the individual level to help us find, and function as, our best selves. First, however, we need to understand why burnout occurs in the first place.

Drivers and Consequences of Burnout

The drivers of burnout vary across specialties, work units, and individuals and have changed as medicine has evolved.[6] Drivers in the modern era include challenges and inefficiencies with the EMR, productivity expectations, frustrations in dealing with health care insurers, availability of resources, and more recently staffing issues as nurses and other professionals have left the field of health care altogether.[7] While these are tangible and obvious drivers of burnout, there are more insidious drivers that are harder to perceive. Critically important is the pervasive epidemic of loneliness and belonging uncertainty we experience in the workplace.[8-10] Studies show that employees who feel lonely, ostracized, and lack a sense of belonging have high rates of job dissatisfaction, decreased job performance, and increased turnover.[11,12] For organizations, focusing on creating belonging leads to a 56% increase in performance, a 50% decrease in turnover, and 75% fewer sick days.[13] This increased engagement saves a 10,000-person company $52 million annually. Belonging is also closely linked to our own sense of personal fulfilment. When we feel we do not belong, we question whether we can be our authentic selves at work, whether we have autonomy, and whether our work is meaningful in a way that matters to us. Decreased perceived autonomy not surprisingly has been strongly linked to burnout.[14]

The consequences of failing to address burnout are costly, not only to health care organizations, but also to individual workers and the patients they care for. Burnout is financially costly through turnover, lost revenue, and employee disengagement, conservatively amounting to $4.6 billion a year in the United States.[15] For individual health care systems, this amounts to $7600/y per employed physician. Individuals who are burned out have higher rates of substance abuse, relationship troubles, depression, and suicide.[16,17] Finally, when physicians are not tending to their own well-being and are burned out, medical errors increase, quality of care suffers, and harm is done to patients.[18-20]

Importance of Well-being and Resilience Training

The opposite of burnout is functioning as our best selves—a level of *full* engagement with our careers and our lives outside of work. The drivers aforementioned are some of the barriers that get in the way of this, along with other non-career-related factors (eg, relationships, financial pressures), and our unique individual traits (eg, genetics, physical and mental health). To provide tools to help us achieve our best selves, the term "Resilience Bank Account" was previously coined by one of the authors (MM) to discuss habits that build resilience and meet challenges we face as individuals.[21] The habits include sleep, exercise, meditation, gratitude, self-compassion, and connection. Here, the authors will once again touch on these important habits, but they will go a step further to discuss the concept of fulfillment and how we can use it to find meaning in the work we do. The authors will also take an in depth look at belonging and discuss the importance of building connection and community.

Training ourselves to be resilient has 2 fundamental purposes. The first is to help us cope and navigate challenges we face as surgeons and humans. This is particularly important in high-stress careers in which we commonly encounter challenges to our resilience—a major complication, the death of a patient, a frequent sense of overwhelm. In addition to building personal resilience, however, we should develop comfort offering peer support to our colleagues who are likely also struggling, which also helps foster a culture of belonging. The second reason to train ourselves to be resilient is as a prophylactic strategy to insulate us against the challenges we will inevitably face that threaten our homeostasis. The first step to create this is to truly understand our motivations, what makes us tick, and what gives meaning to our work. Though sounding simple, it is anything but.

Strategy #1: Start with Fulfillment

In their book *Dark Horse,* Todd Rose and Ogi Ogas describe the concept of the standardization covenant, which promises us—if we only put our heads down, do what is asked of us, and stay the course—that success, as measured by finances and "status," will be the end rewards. [22] As surgeons, we know this covenant well, and indeed, like pilots and the military, society necessarily has a vested interest in the production of highly competent surgeons. But if the true goal of a career is fulfillment, the covenant often fails. The reason is simple: success and fulfillment are 2 distinct entities and are not inextricably linked. Success comes from achieving some predetermined end goal, often by adhering to the covenant's dogma, as demonstrated by the stepwise pathway to becoming a cardiothoracic surgeon. Although this measure of "success" leads to fulfillment for some individuals, it does not guarantee it. While success is seen and bestowed upon us from outside observers, fulfillment is a deeply individual phenomenon and can only be bestowed upon us by ourselves. Fulfillment derives exclusively from the sense that our lives are meaningful.

The fundamental problem with the standardization covenant is that our paths are chosen for us; we are seldom encouraged to ask, "What do I really want?" or, "What truly fulfills me?" While the

standardization covenant works for some, for many it leads to a path of disappointment, frustration, even misery, leaving us with the question, "Whose life am I living?" As Rose and Ogas point out, the only sure path to fulfillment is to abandon the standardization covenant and *start* with fulfillment. Rather than the promised endgame, fulfillment becomes a guiding light. The authors offer 4 suggestions: (1) Know our micromotives (things that inherently drive us and bring us innate energy), (2) Engineer our choices around our micromotives, (3) Wisely choose the strategies we embark on, and (4) Ignore the destination. Ignoring the destination is not something we are often told to do. We are frequently asked, "Where do you see yourself in 10 years?," as if a perfectly manicured path to the top of the standardization covenant is a requisite to future success. As psychologist and Auschwitz survivor, Viktor Frankl suggests in his book *Man's Search for Meaning,* "Don't aim at success—the more you aim at it and make it a target, the more you are going to miss it. For success, like happiness, cannot be pursued; it must ensue…as the unintended side-effect of one's personal dedication to a course greater than oneself. [23]"

Fulfillment is a uniquely individual concept, based on our unique genes, 100 trillion unique neural connections, and our experiences. [24] For all professionals, fulfillment is critically important, and lack of fulfillment is closely linked to burnout.[25] Conversely, fulfillment, and the autonomy to pursue it, is fundamental to our well-being and insulates us from burnout. Tait Shanafelt's group demonstrated this when they surveyed physicians at Mayo Clinic asking respondents which part of their jobs most fulfilled them. [26] They then determined how each person spent their time. Incongruence between fulfilling activities and actual work effort was a highly significant predictor of burnout. The "magic number" seems to be around 20%. Physicians who spent 20% of their time engaged in meaningful, fulfilling activities had significantly decreased burnout and, interestingly, spending more than 20% did not provide an extra boost. [26] Of course, there are things our jobs require that will not fulfill us—documenting in the EMR, participating in meetings that move the hospital's mission forward but do little for our own interests. While we may find ways to lessen these burdens, we will never spend all our time doing meaningful work. The great news is we do not have to.

Taken together, *Dark Horse* and the Mayo Clinic study emphasize that to be our best selves we must both know what fulfills us and have the autonomy to engineer our careers around that fulfillment. But how do we *know* what fulfills us? This can be challenging for those of us who have spent most of our lives embracing the standardization covenant. Marcus Buckingham, in his book *Love + Work,* takes on this important question. [25] Buckingham introduces readers to a Norse term—"*wyrd*"—which can be loosely defined as our guiding spirit, innate to every individual, informed by our unique genetics and circumstances. Understanding our *wyrd* can be challenging but Buckingham offers us some useful tools to do so. Being cognizant of the things to which we purposefully direct our attention, listening to our instincts (ie, the things we inherently enjoy doing), and looking out for moments of flow are important. Flow is a critical concept, coined by Mihaly Csikszentmihalyi, defined as "a state in which people are so involved in an activity that nothing else seems to matter; the experience is so enjoyable that people will continue to do it even at great cost, for the sheer sake of doing it. [27]" Flow has been studied extensively and not surprisingly has important connections to burnout. Achieving flow is protective against burnout, and burnout itself inhibits our ability to achieve flow. [28] In *Love +* Work, Buckingham encourages us to explore this by asking ourselves questions such as "When did I last lose track of time?", "When was I the only person to notice something?", or "When did I want an activity to never end? [24]" When thoughtfully answered, these become useful clues that can guide us to what matters. Buckingham emphasizes that when answering questions, the details matter. When we reflect on what we enjoy it is not simply enough to say, "I love [teaching/research/operating]." We need to dive into the details: Who, what, when, where, and how do I love [teaching/researching/operating]? For example, a person may love teaching an experienced, technically skilled resident a new challenging skill in a one-on-one setting, but that same individual may loathe the opportunity to deliver a didactic lecture on cardiac physiology to a group of first year medical students. Knowing the details should inform the opportunities we seek and help us engineer a path toward fulfillment.

As we better understand ourselves and what fulfills us, the next step is ensuring that we are actually doing those things. For many, this can be hard, especially if we are in a job misaligned with what gives us meaning. Ideally, knowing what fulfills us, we will have negotiated a job that includes protected time (ideally 20%) to engage in those activities. In the common scenario, however, where there is incongruence between fulfillment and actual workflow, there are solutions. The first is we can have an honest conversation with our chair/chief about the incongruence and renegotiate protected time to engage in fulfilling opportunities. Depending on your relationship, departmental/institutional needs, and other factors, this may or may not be successful. A second solution involves pursuing meaningful activities in addition to our routine work on our own time. While this may add to an already full workload (and long-term may create burnout), this has some advantages. By trying a new activity that adds meaning in small time chunks, we gain data on whether it is something we truly love. If we find fulfillment and achieve success in a way that adds value, we can then approach our boss with clout to better negotiate protected time. We may even find our work has already been noticed as valuable without effort. A third option, challenging for many of us, is to simply say "no" to the relative value unit (RVU) and money "carrots"—perhaps not entirely—to give ourselves space and time to pursue meaningful work. And finally, if completely thwarted in our ability to pursue meaningful work, we can move on to another opportunity.

Fulfillment is so fundamentally important to our happiness, well-being, and ability to function as our best selves that it cannot be ignored without serious consequences. If we fail to pursue activities that fulfill us at work, we embark on one of the surest paths to burnout and unhappiness. We simply cannot thrive over the long term. As humans however, we need more than fulfillment to be our best selves. We need to be fulfilled in an environment where we feel connected to others and in which we belong.

Strategy #2: Cultivate Community, Connection, and Belonging

Humans are fundamentally social beings. It is inherent in our evolution, programmed into our genetic code, and manifested in our neurodevelopment. [29,30] Tens of thousands of years ago, we outsurvived our closest relatives, Neanderthals, not because we were physically stronger or possessed larger brains (neither of which is true), but because we underwent a cognitive revolution, informed by our genetics, during which we mastered the ability to work together in tribes. [31] These tribes proved to be more resilient to stresses compared to smaller family units of Neanderthals. Consequently, as tribes became an important survival mechanism for early humans, belonging became a physiologic imperative. The need for connection is so important for humans that our brains have evolved to interpret loneliness and lack of belonging as *pain*, identical to the way we interpret actual physical harm. [32]

Neurologically, our interpretation of threats—whether physical or belonging threats—is governed by the limbic system, centered around the amygdala, often described as our "fight or flight" mechanism. When confronting a threat, our limbic system activates, triggering a physiologic response designed to help us deal with the situation: tachycardia, increased blood flow to the brain and muscles, and a rise in blood glucose levels. While in the short term, this is helpful and protective, chronic exposure to fear-inducing threats leads to significant harm, with increased levels of stress hormones such as cortisol, and decreased heart rate variability. [33] The downstream effects put us at increased risk of diabetes, heart disease, depression, post-traumatic stress disorder, and early mortality. [34–37]

Unfortunately, as complex as our brains have evolved to be, from a physiologic standpoint, we poorly distinguish between physical and emotional threats. The term "belonging uncertainty" was first coined by Gregory Walton and Geoffrey Cohen [38] and refers to "a state of mind in which one suffers from doubts about whether one is fully accepted in a particular environment or ever could be. [39]" As Cohen points out in his book, *Belonging*, when we have belonging uncertainty, we are more sensitive to failure, stop taking risks, see others as threats, and feel misunderstood by those around us. [39] The consequences are profound. Feelings of loneliness or lacking belonging are linked to depression, poor sleep, impaired cognition, cardiovascular disease, poor immune function, and early mortality. [40] The effect on life expectancy for those lacking strong social connections and experiencing loneliness is the equivalent of smoking 15 cigarettes daily. [41] In surgical residents, lack of belonging is strongly correlated with burnout [42,43] and attrition. [44] The loss of social connection has been demonstrated as one of the most significant factors contributing to burnout among physicians. [45] The human brain is not naturally resilient when it comes to belonging uncertainty. It takes very few signals—a comment, a questioning glance, gossip—to make us doubt belonging, while it takes frequent and repeated signals to convince us otherwise. The great thing is that while belonging uncertainty is harmful, cultivating it makes us incredibly resilient to other stresses.

How then can we cultivate belonging in our workplaces? The first step relates back to the concept of fulfillment. By understanding who we are and what fulfills us, we are able express ourselves authentically. This authenticity is a fundamental requirement to building connection with others. [46] Trying to belong to a group without being our authentic selves is not really *belonging* at all: it is *fitting in*, and we and others recognize this as fake. Beyond authenticity, we must build social connections with others. There are many behaviors that help toward that end: exhibiting prosocial behavior, embracing vulnerability, building trust, cultivating psychological safety in our teams, and expressing gratitude.

Exhibiting prosocial behavior achieves 2 important results. First, it increases our own positive emotions. Second, and more importantly for building connection, it increases positive emotions in others and has a metastatic effect. [47] Sigal Barksdale pioneered work on this latter concept, coining the term "emotional contagion." She demonstrated that emotions, both positive and negative have profound effects on groups. In her landmark study published in 2002, [48] groups unknowingly exposed to positive emotional contagion experienced more positive moods and demonstrated better cooperation, decreased interpersonal conflicts, and performed better than groups "infected" by negative contagions. Expression of positive emotions at work has a ripple effect, elevating the moods of those around us and achieving this is remarkably simple: a smile, a warm "hello," offering a compliment, and demonstrating genuine interest in a colleague.

Another way to cultivate belonging is to embrace vulnerability. Historically, vulnerability has wrongly been associated with weakness and is usually avoided. This is especially true for surgeons, who are dogmatically trained to believe that perfection is more than a goal: it is expected. As surgeons, we are taught to pretend we are strong and capable, even when we are not. Because of negative connotations, we limit our vulnerability within our groups, believing we will be shunned. However, this could not be further from the truth. Vulnerability, when used appropriately, has the opposite effect, fostering stronger connections with those around us. Like prosocial behavior, vulnerability has a way of disseminating; once we take off our proverbial masks, others do the same. Brené Brown has studied vulnerability in leaders for decades, arguing convincingly that it is a requisite for leaders to be most effective. [49] Vulnerability, she notes, does not require disclosure of our most personal details to our colleagues, but does require us to have the courage to allow others to see us as our true selves so they can be comfortable being seen as theirs. Vulnerability is essential for meaningful connection.

Like vulnerability, trust encourages belonging and lies at the heart of all relationships. We are less willing to connect with others without trusting them, and once trust is breached, we become reluctant to reengage. Put simply, without trust, meaningful relationships do not materialize. Trust is something we intuitively feel, yet is challenging to identify the individual components comprising it. David Maister, in his book, *The Trusted Advisor,* created a trust equation with 4 components: *Trust = (Credibility + Reliability + Intimacy)/Self-Orientation.* [50] We can use this tool to evaluate how trustworthy others see us. According to Maister's coauthor Charles Green, of all the trust equation components, intimacy is the most important. Intimacy is related to the quality of relationships we nurture with those around us and is surprisingly easy to cultivate. Getting to know our colleagues, showing them that we care about them in a genuine way establishes intimacy. To do so requires vulnerability, empathy, and sincere curiosity. The denominator of the equation, self-orientation, defined as how much we put our own interests ahead of others, negatively detracts from trust. When we are self-orientated, others mistrust our intentions and are reluctant to build relationships. If we want to build trust and connect with others, we must check our egos at the door, give our attention to others, and engage with our teams without distraction.

As surgeons, we frequently work within high-performance teams, groups of people working closely together with shared purpose, vision, and goals. High-performance teams take on challenging tasks to achieve something meaningful that cannot be accomplished individually. Members of high-performance teams report an increased sense of belonging, just as belonging itself is a critical element of a high-performance team. [51] As surgeons, we have the daily opportunity to be a part of such teams and to lead them, inside and out of the operating room. There are many things we can do as leaders to foster and build this collaborative teamwork. Amy Edmondson, author of *The Fearless Organization* and a leading expert on psychological safety, stresses the importance of leaders creating psychologically safe environments where people thrive together. Edmondson defines psychological safety as "a climate in which people are comfortable expressing and being themselves" and "feel comfortable sharing concerns and mistakes without fear of embarrassment or retribution. [52]" Edmondson identifies ways that we can cultivate psychological safety within our teams including: (1) Ensuring alignment of the vision and goals, (2) Encouraging participation from all team members, (3) Showing gratitude for the courage of speaking up. The leader of the team is most responsible for creating an atmosphere where psychological safety thrives. The end result is deep connection and a strong sense of belonging.

Finally, gratitude is an effective way to cultivate belonging. Gratitude negatively correlates with loneliness and powerfully moderates feelings of belonging and connection. [53] Gratitude connects us with others and builds our individual resilience. Gratitude stimulates endogenous opioid pathways and releases oxytocin, a "feel good" hormone."[54] There are several techniques to practice gratitude, including increasing our conscious awareness of people and things for which we are grateful, keeping a gratitude journal, or actively expressing gratitude to others either through writing or conversationally. [21] Regardless of the technique, gratitude is inextricably connected to our own well-being. [55] Directly expressing gratitude to others, however, has the obvious benefit of also increasing the well-being of the recipient, fostering belonging.

Belonging is critically important to our well-being, decreases burnout, and increases our personal resilience. This was nicely demonstrated in a study recently published, where physicians were randomized to a belonging intervention or a noninterventional control. [56] The physicians in the intervention arm met in small groups centered around reflection, discussion of shared experiences, and a meal. Those that were part of these Colleagues Meeting to Promote and Sustain Satisfaction (COMPASS) groups demonstrated a 12.7% decrease in burnout, compared to a 1.9% increase in the controls. The intervention group experienced less depression and were less likely to leave their current practice. This low-cost intervention is a simple way to promote belonging at our institutions. Other examples we have successfully enacted are book clubs centered around wellness and resilience, and storytelling sessions, where clinicians gather to talk and listen.

Strategy #3: Mitigate Microstresses and Avoid Overwhelm

It is easy to appreciate *macro*stresses we encounter in our lives: the death of a close friend, a seriously ill family member, a bad outcome on a patient on whom we have operated. These can unravel us in not-so-subtle ways. Dealing with these macrostresses is important for our overall well-being and depending on the nature and severity of the stress, may necessitate peer coaching, professional therapy, taking time away from work, or a host of other interventions to get us back on track. However, a slower and more insidious unraveling occurs with the *microstresses* we experience daily. Rob Cross and Karen Dillon, in their book *The Microstress Effect,* define microstresses as "tiny moments of stress triggered by people in our personal and professional lives; stresses so routine that we barely register them but whose cumulative toll is debilitating. [57]" Microstresses cannot be avoided since they are unintentionally caused by the people we spend the vast majority our time with: our families, friends, and colleagues. There are countless examples of the microstresses we may experience as surgeons: a friend reaches out with a problem as we are getting ready to scrub into a case; our child comes to us in tears because she did not make the school basketball team as we are working on a manuscript; while already stretched thin, our emails add endless new tasks to our plates. Cross and Dillon classify the microstresses that we experience into 3 categories: those that drain our capacity, those that deplete us emotionally, and those that challenge our identity. Microstresses have troubling long-term effects on our health and well-being, contributing to chronic diseases like hypertension and affect us hormonally and metabolically. When not effectively dealing with microstresses, they affect our ability to concentrate, problem-solve, and be at our best selves.

There are plenty of ways to mitigate microstresses by subtly or not-so-subtly pushing back against them. One method that has worked for both authors of this article is removal of email applications from our phones. This decreases the constant demands for our attention by the small, buzzing devices we all carry in our pockets. Instead, we set time aside twice daily to respond to emails in a focused manner. Another very important way to mitigate microstress is to live our lives more intentionally. This means making decisions with purpose, aligning our actions with our personal goals and values. Not only does intentional living increase personal resilience, but it insulates us against the microstresses we face, allowing us to set better boundaries. A final suggestion is to spend time with others building meaningful connections, especially when there is a focus on boosting resilience, physical well-being, and engineering a sense of purpose. It is important to build a network of people we can authentically connect with, lean on for support, and reciprocate with our own empathy.

Despite best intentions, we are bound to feel overwhelmed at times for reasons often under our control, but sometimes not. Microstresses contribute to feelings of overwhelm, but so do many other things: overextending ourselves by agreeing to things that deplete our time and energy and do not fulfill us, the sheer amount of work combined with our responsibilities as a parent or spouse, an increase in workload due to a partner on long-term sick leave. Strategies to avoid these situations are critical, such as saying "no" to opportunities misaligned with the intentional life we want to live. But sometimes avoidance strategies are not enough. Mindfulness meditation is one way to accept and cope with feelings of overwhelm. Mindfulness mediation, one of many meditative practices, focuses the attention on the breath and upon noticing the mind wandering (as it often does), redirects attention back to the breath. [58] The skill honed here is redirection of the mind, nonjudgmental acceptance of distracting thoughts, and the ability to let them go. To put this in context of overwhelm, mindfulness meditation trains us to accept these feelings without judgment, anchoring us to the present. Physiologically, much happens when we meditate: our sympathetic nervous systems quiet in favor of a calming parasympathetic response, [59] blood pressure and heart rate decrease, heart rate variability increases, [60] and the body's cortisol response diminishes. [61] Devoting just 10 minutes daily to this practice is enough to achieve many of its benefits and is feasible even for busy clinicians.

Strategy #4: Build a Resilience Bank Account

As emphasized in "The Resilience Bank Account: Skills for Optimal Performance," our ability to show up as our best selves is influenced by 3 domains: daily cumulative stress from our busy lives at work and home, external events that happen to us, and our personal skills and attributes that inform how easily we can adapt to challenges. [21] Like building a muscle by regularly going to the gym, our resilience can be strengthened by training, increasing the "assets" of our resilience bank accounts. Many of the strategies aforementioned, such as building connection, expressing gratitude, and meditating, are ways we can do this. In addition, sleep and exercise are 2 other critical ways to increase our personal resilience.

While insufficient sleep is a problem for many, it is especially problematic for surgeons, who not only have frequent sleep disruptions due to on-call emergencies but are trained in a culture that values the ability to deal sleep loss as an important asset and rite of passage. The importance of sleep is well understood. While person to person variations exist, most adult humans need 7 to 9 hours of sleep nightly. [62] Chronically, curtailing sleep is problematic, especially because rapid eye movement (REM) sleep is disproportionately affected. REM sleep, which occurs more frequently toward the end of the sleep cycle, is important for processing information and experiences and regulates our moods and emotions. [63] For surgeons, sleep deprivation decreases performance on high-level cognitive tasks [64] and while no studies conclusively suggest sleep deprivation affects technical abilities, there is little doubt it affects our moods and well-being. Losing sleep for several nights in a row amplifies the consequences, creating a debt which must be repaid. Insufficient sleep has tremendous consequences to our physical and mental health, including a 12% increase in all-cause mortality, [65] increased cardiovascular disease, obesity, metabolic syndrome, depression, anxiety, and dementia. [66,67] The other insidious consequence of insufficient sleep is impairment of our ability to sustain healthy relationships with our colleagues and families. When sleep deprived, our capacity for patience and grace toward others decreases, our sense of belonging decreases, with tremendous consequences.

We are aware of the health benefits of exercise, including its prevention of heart disease, hypertension, diabetes, and metabolic syndrome. Exercise, however, is a powerful tool not only for physical, but also for mental health. Exercise decreases the incidence of depression by 17% to 41% [68] and a meta-analysis demonstrated exercise as a potent treatment for depression. [69] The proposed mechanisms include myokine release, decreased inflammatory and oxidative stress markers such as IL-6, and increased levels of brain-derived neurotrophic factor (BDNF). [70] Exercise-triggered BDNF release leads to increased brain plasticity and an increase in volume of the hippocampus, a part of the brain important for learning, memory, and emotion. Exercise increases our ability to think creatively, improves sleep quality, and improves our mood. Exercise can be a valuable way to make and strengthen connections with others and create belonging.

As surgeons, we encounter many barriers to exercise, most of which are fabricated excuses: lack of time, energy, or ability; we have other priorities, or a perception that spending time on ourselves through exercise is overindulgent in the face of our other responsibilities. The fact is that these are largely untrue. There are many practical ways to build exercise into an already busy routine. First, like any commitment we care about, we can put exercise on our calendars. Treating exercise like a "meeting" or "protected time" is a good way to start. We can also build exercise and movement into our daily routines. Taking a 15-min walk in the middle of a workday, between operating room cases, or between clinic patients is feasible for many and can impact our well-being. When meeting with a small group, consider scheduling a "walking meeting," outside, if possible. Because exercise promotes critical thinking and creativity, it may be surprising how problem solving increases during such a meeting.

SUMMARY

As surgeons, we have a lot on our plates, and considering the fact that most of us are also parents, spouses, friends, and community members, it is easy to feel the pressures of work and life cumulatively combine, becoming intensely stressful. This stress detracts from our ability to be our best selves. Training ourselves to be more resilient in the face of these stresses is paramount to functioning as our best selves and living more fulfilling lives. Beginning with fulfillment, cultivating connection and belonging, mitigating microstresses, avoiding a sense of overwhelm, and making frequent deposits into our resilience bank accounts will help us do just that. We owe it to our patients and our families, but most importantly we owe this to ourselves.

CLINICS CARE POINTS

- Spending 20% of our time on meaningful and fulfilling activities is associated with decreased burnout and increased well-being.
- Connection and belonging have profound effects on our mental and physical health.
- Building healthy habits into our schedules: adequate sleep, exercise, meditation, for instance, improve our personal resilience.

DISCLOSURE

The authors have no disclosures.

REFERENCES

1. Shanafelt TD, West CP, Dyrbye LN, et al. Changes in burnout and satisfaction with work-life integration in physicians during the first 2 years of the COVID-19 pandemic. Mayo Clin Proc 2022;97:2248–58.
2. Shanafelt TD, Balch CM, Bechamps GJ, et al. Burnout and career satisfaction among american surgeons. Trans Meet Am Surg Assoc 2009;127:107–15.
3. Bremner RM, Ungerleider RM, Ungerleider J, et al. Well-being of cardiothoracic surgeons in the time of COVID-19: a survey by the wellness committee of the american association for thoracic surgery. Semin Thorac Cardiovasc Surg 2022. https://doi.org/10.1053/j.semtcvs.2022.10.002.
4. Dyrbye LN, West CP, Satele D, et al. Burnout among U.S. medical students, residents, and early career physicians relative to the general U.S. population. Acad Med 2014;89:443–51.

5. Chow OS, Sudarshan M, Maxfield MW, et al. National survey of burnout and distress among cardiothoracic surgery trainees. Ann Thorac Surg 2021; 111:2066–71.

6. Pangallo A, Atwell T, Roe K, et al. Understanding modern drivers of the employee experience in healthcare. Patient Experience Journal 2022;9:46–61.

7. West CP, Dyrbye LN, Shanafelt TD. Physician burnout: contributors, consequences and solutions. J Intern Med 2018;283:516–29.

8. Lin SH, Huang YC. Investigating the relationships between loneliness and learning burnout. Act Learn High Educ 2012;13:231–43.

9. Wood RE, Brown RE, Kinser PA. The connection between loneliness and burnout in nurses: an integrative review. Appl Nurs Res 2022;66.

10. Rogers E, Polonijo AN, Carpiano RM. Getting by with a little help from friends and colleagues: testing how residents' social support networks affect loneliness and burnout. Can Fam Physician 2016;62:e677–83.

11. Li M, Xu X, Kwan HK. Consequences of workplace ostracism: a meta-analytic review. Front Psychol 2021;12:1–14.

12. Schaechter JD, Goldstein R, Zafonte RD, et al. Workplace belonging of women healthcare professionals relates to likelihood of leaving. J Healthc Leader 2023;15:273–84.

13. Carr EW. The value of belonging at work. Harv Bus Rev 2019.

14. Fernet C, Austin S, Trépanier S-G, et al. How do job characteristics contribute to burnout? exploring the distinct mediating roles of perceived autonomy, competence, and relatedness. Eur J Work Organ Psychol 2013;22:123–37.

15. Han S, Shanafelt TD, Sinsky CA, et al. Estimating the attributable cost of physician burnout in the United States. Ann Intern Med 2019;170:784.

16. Koutsimani P, Montgomery A, Georganta K. The relationship between burnout, depression, and anxiety: a systematic review and meta-analysis. Front Psychol 2019;10:284.

17. Fitzpatrick O, Biesma R, Conroy RM, et al. Prevalence and relationship between burnout and depression in our future doctors: a cross-sectional study in a cohort of preclinical and clinical medical students in Ireland. BMJ Open 2019;9:e023297.

18. Salyers MP, Bonfils KA, Luther L, et al. The relationship between professional burnout and quality and safety in healthcare: a meta-analysis. J Gen Intern Med 2017;32:475–82.

19. Tawfik DS, Scheid A, Profit J, et al. Evidence relating health care provider burnout and quality of care: a systematic review and meta-analysis. Ann Intern Med 2019;171:555.

20. Montgomery A, Todorova I, Baban A, et al. Improving quality and safety in the hospital: The link between organizational culture, burnout, and quality of care. Br J Health Psychol 2013;18: 656–62.

21. Maddaus M. The resilience bank account: skills for optimal performance. Ann Thorac Surg 2020;109: 18–25.

22. Rose T, Dark Horse O. Achieving success through the pursuit of fulfillment. 1st edition. New York, (NY): HarperOne, an imprint of HarperCollins Publishers; 2018.

23. Frankl VE. Man's search for meaning : an introduction to logotherapy. Boston, (MA): Beacon Press; 1962.

24. Buckingham M. Love + work: how to find what you love, love what you do, and do it for the rest of your life. 1st edition. Boston, (MA): Harvard Business Review Press; 2022.

25. Prentice S, Elliott T, Dorstyn D, et al. Burnout, well-being and how they relate: A qualitative study in general practice trainees. Med Educ 2023;57: 243–55.

26. Shanafelt TD, West CP, Sloan JA, et al. Career fit and burnout among academic faculty. Arch Intern Med 2009;169:990–5.

27. Csikszentmihalyi M. Flow: the psychology of optimal experience. 1st edition. New York, NY: HarperCollins Publishers; 1990.

28. Aust F, Beneke T, Peifer C, et al. The relationship between flow experience and burnout symptoms: a systematic review. Int J Environ Res Publ Health 2022;19:3865.

29. Ebstein RP, Israel S, Chew SH, et al. Genetics of human social behavior. Neuron 2010;65:831–44.

30. Baumeister RF, Leary MR. The need to belong: desire for interpersonal attachments as a fundamental human emotion. Psychol Bull 1995;117: 497–529.

31. Harari YN. Sapiens: a brief history of humankind. New York, NY: HarperCollins Publishers; 2015.

32. Eisenberger NI, Lieberman MD. Why rejection hurts: a common neural alarm system for physical and social pain. Trends Cognit Sci 2004;8: 294–300.

33. Kim H-G, Cheon E-J, Bai D-S, et al. Stress and heart rate variability: a meta-analysis and review of the literature. Psychiatry Investig 2018;15:235–45.

34. Satyjeet F, Naz S, Kumar V, et al. Psychological stress as a risk factor for cardiovascular disease: a case-control study. Cureus 2020;12:e10757.

35. Sharma VK, Singh TG. Chronic stress and diabetes mellitus: interwoven pathologies. Curr Diabetes Rev 2020;16:546–56.

36. Tafet GE, Bernardini R. Psychoneuroendocrinological links between chronic stress and depression. Prog Neuro-Psychopharmacol Biol Psychiatry 2003;27:893–903.

37. Eplov LF, Jørgensen T, Birket-Smith M, et al. Mental vulnerability as a predictor of early mortality. Epidemiology 2005;16:226–32.

38. Walton GM, Cohen GL. A Question of belonging: race, social fit, and achievement. J Pers Soc Psychol 2007;92:82–96.

39. Cohen GL Belonging. The science of creating connection and bridging divides. 1st edition. New York, (NY): W.W. Norton and Company, Inc; 2022.

40. Hawkley LC, Capitanio JP. Perceived social isolation, evolutionary fitness and health outcomes: a lifespan approach. Philos. Trans. R. Soc. B: Biol Sci 2015;370:20140114.

41. Holt-Lunstad J, Smith TB, Layton JB. Social relationships and mortality risk: a meta-analytic review. PLoS Med 2010;7:e1000316.

42. Puranitee P, Kaewpila W, Heeneman S, et al. Promoting a sense of belonging, engagement, and collegiality to reduce burnout: a mixed methods study among undergraduate medical students in a non-Western, Asian context. BMC Med Educ 2022;22:327.

43. Aker S, Şahin MK. The relationship between school burnout, sense of school belonging and academic achievement in preclinical medical students. Adv Health Sci Educ Theory Pract 2022;27(4):949–63.

44. Salles A, Wright RC, Milam L, et al. Social belonging as a predictor of surgical resident well-being and attrition. J Surg Educ 2019;76:370–7.

45. Southwick SM, Southwick FS. The loss of social connectedness as a major contributor to physician burnout. JAMA Psychiatr 2020;77:449–50.

46. Menzies D, Davidson B. Authenticity and belonging: the experience of being known in the group. Group Anal 2002;35(1):43–55.

47. Berinato S. What do we know about loneliness and work? Harv Bus Rev 2017;28.

48. Barsade SG. The ripple effect: emotional contagion and its influence on group behavior. Adminstrative Science Quarterly 2002;47:644–75.

49. Brown B. Daring greatly: how the courage to be vulnerable transforms the way we live, love, parent, and lead. 1st edition. New York, NY: Gotham Books; 2012.

50. Maister DH, Galford R, Green C. The trusted advisor. New York, NY: Simon & Schuster; 2001.

51. Robbins M. We're all in this together: creating a team culture of high performance, trust, and belonging. 1st edition. Carlsbad, CA: Hay House, Inc.; 2020.

52. Edmondson AC. The fearless organization: creating psychological safety in the workplace for learning, innovation, and growth. First edition. Hoboken, NJ: John Wiley and Sons, Inc.; 2019.

53. Caputo A. The relationship between gratitude and loneliness: the potential benefits of gratitude for promoting social bonds. Eur J Psychol 2015;11:323–34.

54. Henning M, Fox GR, Kaplan J, et al. A potential role for mu-opioids in mediating the positive effects of gratitude. Front Psychol 2017;8:868.

55. Wood AM, Froh JJ, Geraghty AWA. Gratitude and well-being: a review and theoretical integration. Clin Psychol Rev 2010;30:890–905.

56. West CP, Dyrbye LN, Satele DV, et al. Colleagues meeting to promote and sustain satisfaction (compass) groups for physician well-being a randomized clinical trial. Mayo Clin Proc 2021;96:2606–14.

57. Cross R, Dillon K. The microstress effect: how little things pile up and create big problems—and what to do about it. 1st edition. Boston, MA: Harvard Business Review Press; 2023.

58. Tan LBG, Lo BCY, Macrae CN. Brief mindfulness meditation improves mental state attribution and empathizing. PLoS One 2014;9:e110510.

59. Tang Y-Y, Ma Y, Fan Y, et al. Central and autonomic nervous system interaction is altered by short-term meditation. Proc Natl Acad Sci USA 2009;106:8865–70.

60. Wu S-D, Lo P-C. Inward-attention meditation increases parasympathetic activity: a study based on heart rate variability. Biomed Res 2008;29:245–50.

61. Turakitwanakan W, Mekseepralard C, Busarakumtragul P. Effects of mindfulness meditation on serum cortisol of medical students. J. Méd. Assoc. Thail. Chotmaihet thangphaet 2013;96(Suppl 1):S90–5.

62. Panel CC, Watson NF, Badr MS, et al. Recommended amount of sleep for a healthy adult: a joint consensus statement of the american academy of sleep medicine and sleep research society. J Clin Sleep Med 2015;11:591–2.

63. Miller KE, Gehrman PR. REM sleep: what is it good for? Curr Biol 2019;29:R806–7.

64. Whelehan DF, Alexander M, Connelly TM, et al. Sleepy surgeons: a multi-method assessment of sleep deprivation and performance in surgery. J Surg Res 2021;268:145–57.

65. Cappuccio FP, D'Elia L, Strazzullo P, et al. Sleep duration and all-cause mortality: a systematic review and meta-analysis of prospective studies. Sleep 2010;33:585–92.

66. Iftikhar IH, Donley MA, Mindel J, et al. Sleep duration and metabolic syndrome. an updated dose–risk metaanalysis. Ann Am Thorac Soc 2015;12:1364–72.

67. Korostovtseva L, Bochkarev M, Sviryaev Y. Sleep and cardiovascular risk. Sleep Med Clin 2021;16:485–97.

68. Schuch FB, Stubbs B. The role of exercise in preventing and treating depression. Curr Sports Med Rep 2019;18:299–304.

69. Schuch FB, Vancampfort D, Richards J, et al. Exercise as a treatment for depression: a meta-analysis adjusting for publication bias. J Psychiatr Res 2016;77:42–51.

70. Pedersen BK. Physical activity and muscle–brain crosstalk. Nat Rev Endocrinol 2019;15:383–92.

Moving?

Make sure your subscription moves with you!

To notify us of your new address, find your **Clinics Account Number** (located on your mailing label above your name), and contact customer service at:

Email: journalscustomerservice-usa@elsevier.com

800-654-2452 (subscribers in the U.S. & Canada)
314-447-8871 (subscribers outside of the U.S. & Canada)

Fax number: 314-447-8029

Elsevier Health Sciences Division
Subscription Customer Service
3251 Riverport Lane
Maryland Heights, MO 63043

ELSEVIER

Printed and bound by CPI Group (UK) Ltd, Croydon, CR0 4YY

08/05/2025

01864751-0014